Encyclopedia of Power Foods for Health and Longer Life

Carlson Wade

Foreword by William S. Keezer, M.D.

Parker Publishing Company, Inc., West Nyack, N.Y.

PARKER PUBLISHING COMPANY, INC.

West Nyack, N.Y.

Reward Edition . . . . . . September 1982

This book is a reference work based on research by the author. The opinions expressed herein are not necessarily those of or endorsed by the publisher. The directions stated in this book are in no way to be considered as a substitute for consultation with a duly licensed doctor.

Librarv of Congress Cataloging in Publication Data

Wade, Carlson.
Encyclopedia of power foods for health and longer life.

Includes bibliographical references and index.
1. Diet therapy. 2. Nutrition. 3. Food, Natural.
I. Title. [DNLM: 1. Diet therapy--Encyclopedias--Popular works. 2. Food--Encyclopedias--Popular works.
WB13 W119a]
RM216.W28 615'.854 79-18250

Printed in the United States of America

DEDICATION

To YOUR better health and longer life

Other books by the author:

Helping Your Health with Enzymes
Magic Minerals: Key to Better Health
The Natural Way to Health Through Controlled Fasting
Carlson Wade's Gourmet Health Foods Cookbook
Natural and Folk Remedies
The Natural Laws of Healthful Living
Health Tonics, Elixirs and Potions for the Look and Feel of Youth
Natural Hormones: The Secret of Youthful Health
Health Secrets from the Orient
Magic Enzymes: Key to Youth and Health
The Miracle of Organic Vitamins for Better Health
Miracle Protein: Secret of Natural Cell-Tissue Rejuvenation
All-Natural Pain Relievers
How to Achieve Fast, Permanent Weight Loss with the New Enzyme-Catalyst Diet
Brand Name Handbook of Protein, Calories and Carbohydrates
Slimfasting—the Quick "Pounds Off" Way to Youthful Slimness
Healing and Revitalizing Your Vital Organs
Miracle Rejuvenation Energizers
Encyclopedia of Power Foods for Health and Longer Life

Foreword by a Doctor of Medicine

The *Encyclopedia of Power Foods for Health and Longer Life* is one of the most important health books you will ever need!

It places right at your fingertips a vast treasure of health-revitalizing and youth-extending programs for every member of the family, no matter what age. Follow these programs in your own home with great ease for speedy results.

Carlson Wade, the leading medical writer and distinguished nutritionist, has created a valuable new guide to the attainment of better health and youthful appearance, and the addition of more productive and energy-filled years to your lifespan.

He shows you how you can easily alert your biological responses and be refreshingly rejuvenated in body and mind. You will be speedily rewarded with more youthful vitality, improved health, longer life. His clearly described step-by-step programs are very simple to follow. They quickly help produce desired "feel better" benefits.

The Encyclopedia of Power Foods for Health and Longer Life will protect you against hundreds of common and uncommon ailments. This volume tells you how to overcome disorders such as allergies, arteriosclerosis, thin blood, respiratory weakness, digestive-intestinal upsets, aging skin, inadequate sight and hearing, and much, much more. You will learn how to solve these problems, how to use ordinary foods and methods to release a "fountain of youth" within your body. You will discover how to multiply your energy, how to roll back the years and make life beautifully youthful again.

Carlson Wade has prepared an extremely valuable program, presented in this up-to-date minute reference book of healing and revitalization of total body and mind. It is the most helpful book on health and longevity I have ever seen. It is just like having a specialist right in your own home. Use it. Enjoy the rewards of being able to look and feel "forever young" in a matter of moments.

William S. Keezer, M.D.

What This Book Will Do for You

Beginning with the very first page, this book will show you:

1. How certain power foods are able to wake up your hidden built-in youth reserves to give you self-rejuvenation from head to toe.
2. How to use everyday power foods to help you get more supercharged joy out of daily living, at home or at work.
3. How these dynamic power foods boost energy, increase vigor, stimulate vitality and activate your internal forces of regeneration.

But this is only a sampling of the benefits now available to you in this valuable one-volume guide to better health and youth restoration.

Within the covers of this all-purpose encyclopedia, you are given hundreds of different power food remedies that speedily correct many, many conditions that may be limiting your enjoyment of youthful good health.

These power foods help reverse the tide of an ailment, then bring about speedy recovery. This collection of "foods that heal" is available for your quick use. They help correct ordinary day-to-day distress symptoms, ease annoying aches, eliminate the problem of premature aging. In short, these power foods create super-health. They alert your sluggish metabolism. They invigorate your sleepy responses. You then bounce back into the mainstream of an active lifestyle.

This one-volume encyclopedia helps everyone who is eager to glow with the joy of everyday living whether at work, at home, at play.

Do you want to discover new worlds of limitless vitality and restored health? Then this book is your passport to a new horizon of eternal youth.

This book is especially helpful for people who may not yet have serious problems. Instead, you have the little everyday symptoms such as a nagging ache, a choking sensation, a vitality drain and less-than-adequate feelings of good health. You may be troubled by creeping body restrictions, limitations of your responses and reflexes. This book will show you how these and other problems can be "washed away" through the use of power foods. These same power foods will help restore biological balance. You will enjoy a feeling of refreshing second youth, often in a little while.

Arranged in 70 sections with hundreds of sub-divisions, this book is easy to read. In terms of symptoms, descriptions, then step-by-step programs, you are able to follow the suggestions to bring about healing in a few moments.

For the first time, you have the answers to hundreds of different everyday problems and their speedy correction. NO drugs. NO devices. NO complications. Many of the programs can be followed in a few moments for quick reward with revitalized good feeling.

Just flip to your selected heading. Look down the pages. In moments, you have the power food healing program at your fingertips. In moments, you can reap the rewards of better health and longer life.

To help enjoy better health and longer life, turn to the first page. The road to super-health lies before you.

Carlson Wade

Table of Contents

ALCOHOLISM
Power foods that help solve drinking problems

You can strengthen your body and mind to resist the drinking urge through the use of a group of wonder foods. These foods help you build strength to overcome the health- and life-draining effects of alcohol. They will not only block the urge to drink, but they will also help restore the bloom of youth to your face, improve the vigor of your internal organs and bring new youthful joy to your life. By using these wonder foods, you will be able to revitalize your entire body from head to toe, inside and outside, so that you will delight in a liquor-free new lifestyle.

Alcoholism: the Health-Destroying Facts. Drinking, no matter how mild or infrequent, creates a sneaky and gradual destruction of your body and mind. Alcohol's first effect on your brain is to slow down the area that controls judgment and thought. It interferes with your normal ability to do everyday mental tasks, to remember, to understand, to reason, to make decisions. Alcohol also slows down the brain area that controls muscular coordination. It interferes with your normal ability to perform simple physical tasks: to coordinate movement of your arms and legs, to speak clearly, to balance yourself.

Even in moderate amounts, alcohol leads to irritation or inflammation of parts of your digestive system; habitual drinking may seriously affect your heart, liver, stomach and other vital organs. In many situations, even a diluted drink or two may cause emotional shock, weight gain from edema (water storage in body cells), serious liver degeneration, heart tissue destruction. It is also the culprit responsible for conditions of high blood pressure, respiratory distress and diabetes, to name just a few of the age-causing reactions that result from this habit. Drinking is also said to reduce your life expectancy and steal at least 15 years from your lifeline. To help stop this thievery, a program of nutritional healing gets to the *cause* of the problem and helps to eliminate the urge to reach for one or more drinks.

The Power Food Method of Reversing Alcoholism. Power foods are able to strengthen segments of the brain which have become distorted or degenerated through alcohol abuse. Alcohol destroys brain cells, weakening the hypothalamus (a portion of the brain involved in appetite control) so that there is an abnormal craving for one drink after another. Power foods are needed to reverse this disturbance in cellular metabolism and invigorate the hypothalamus so that there is a gradual reduction in the physiological derangement involved in the drinking urge. With a properly nourished hypothalamus, there is a gradual reduction and eventual reversal of the alcoholism urge.

A POWER FOOD FORMULA FOR CONTROLLING AND ENDING ALCOHOLISM

A combination of nutrients can restore and rebuild the hypothalamus and create both a control and end of the alcohol problem. This power food formula, created by nutritional scientist Dr. Roger J. Williams,[1] consists of nutrients in a special blend that work cooperatively to boost youthful cell-tissue-molecular restoration so that your hypothalamus and other brain segments can resist the urge to drink.

Where to Get This Power Food Formula. Take a copy of this power food formula to any pharmacy or health food store and ask for a supply to be made to these specifications. You take one tablet or capsule daily. Here is the power food formula to control and end alcoholism as created by Dr. Williams in his laboratory:

[1]*Alcoholism, the Nutritional Approach*, by Roger J. Williams, Ph.D., University of Texas Press, Austin, Texas, 1959.

Vitamins

Vitamin A	20,000 international units
Vitamin D	1,000 international units
Vitamin C (ascorbic acid)	200 milligrams
Vitamin B_1 (thiamine)	4 milligrams
Vitamin B_2 (riboflavin)	4 milligrams
Vitamin B_6 (pyridoxine)	6 milligrams
Niacinamide	40 milligrams
Pantothenate	40 milligrams
Vitamin B_{12}	10 micrograms
Inositol	200 milligrams
Choline	200 milligrams
Vitamin E (tocopherol)	200 units

Minerals

Calcium	300 milligrams
Phosphorus	250 milligrams
Magnesium	100 milligrams
Copper	1 milligram
Iodine	0.1 milligram
Iron	10 milligrams
Maganese	1 milligram
Zinc	5 milligrams

Power Food Formula Benefits: Taking one tablet a day reportedly will improve the molecular biological process so that cells and tissues become repaired. The hypothalamus, particularly, responds to this formula, and its components, formerly ravaged or degenerated through the corrosive action of alcohol, now become revived and renewed. Strengthened, it controls the appetite for drink and helps solve this health program.

Power Food Ends Drinking Urge in 30 Days. Ronald M., taking this power food formula for just 30 days, reported that he no longer had a craving for whiskey. It helped end his drinking problem!

Free of Compulsive Drinking. This power food formula was given to the drinking husband of Susan A. In a short while, he was free of his formerly compulsive drinking desire. Susan A. says that her drinking husband remained free of this habit even after five years!

Helps Control Periodic Drinking Urge. Each morning, Edith L. secretly "spiked" her husband's breakfast tomato juice with this power food formula. He had a history of drinking over 20 years. "I would never have believed that it could help my husband," says Edith L., after seeing how this formula controlled his drinking urge.

Drinking Problem Solved. Bernice H. was married to a drinking husband. He would consume about 26 ounces (nearly a full quart!) every single day for nearly ten years. He tried the group therapy associations with no success. Bernice H. says, "My husband tried the power food formula with immediate success. Within a couple of months, he was completely cured. He has not had a single relapse!"

Herbal Power Food for Alcohol Control. Angelica root or leaves taken as a tea is said to help block the urge to drink more alcohol. It contains the amino acid, glutamine, which is able to nourish the brain and stabilize the appestat mechanism to block the urge for consumption of alcohol. It also helps protect brain and body cells and tissues against serious alcoholic poisoning. Angelica root or leaves may be brewed as a tea. Just add one teaspoon of this herb to one cup of freshly boiled water. Flavor with some lemon or lime juice and a bit of honey. Drink three cups per day. This herb is available at almost all health stores as well as herbal pharmacies.

Whole Grains Provide Power Food Vitamin for Alcohol Solution. Fresh whole grains in the form of wheat germ, bran and brewer's yeast, as well as breads, rolls, muffins and cereals are a treasure of the B-complex vitamins needed to solve the drinking problem. Use these power foods daily to help turn the tide in the drinking urge.

Benefit: Since alcohol is high in carbohydrates (but totally void of vitamins), your body finds it difficult to utilize these sugars and starches. It must draw on your B-complex supplies for carbohydrate metabolization. This now leads to emotional upsets and a weakness that is transformed into a craving for more alcoholic stabilization.

Reverse this tide by boosting your supplies of B-complex vitamins to avoid depletion and to help increase your power to resist alcohol. Add wheat germs, bran and brewer's yeast to baking, cereals, stews, casseroles and soups. Mix in any fruit or vegetable juice. Blenderize for a minute and you'll have a tasty and alcohol-fighting power beverage! It works speedily in repairing your metabolic network and helping your body solve the craving for drink.

See Dizziness, Fatigue, Liver, Low Blood Sugar.

ALLERGIES
Power foods that ease-relieve-eliminate allergic conditions

An allergy is a condition of unusual reaction to substances ordinarily harmless. These substances may be taken into your body by being inhaled or swallowed or by contact with your skin. They may come from an infection in your body. These sensitizing substances that cause a reaction are called *allergens*.

Common allergens that cause unpleasant reactions ranging from sniffling to respiratory congestion and from skin outbreak to gastro-intestinal upheaval include: pollens, molds, house dust, animal danders (skin shed by dogs, cats, horses, rabbits), feathers (from pillows), cornstarch and gums in certain foods, kapok (silky fibers used as mattress fillings or for insulation), wool, cottonseed. Others include dyes, perfumes, metals, chemicals, medicines, insect stings, temperature extremes, as well as bacteria and viruses. Sensitivity may not appear at first contact, but may develop after repeated exposure.

Neglected, an allergy worsens as symptoms become more severe. Weakening of the respiratory-digestive tract renders it sensitive to other assaults. This causes a drain on your basic health. While an allergy in itself may not be considered fatal, it can so upset your vital organs that they become impaired in function and you may find you have a reduced life expectancy along with premature aging. Constant sneezing, wheezing and coughing siphon off important energy and hasten the onset of debilitation and deterioration of cells, tissues and major (and minor) organs. Correct the *cause* of your allergy and your body will respond with better health and a longer, more joyful lifespan.

THE EVERYDAY POWER FOOD THAT IS A NATURAL ANTIBIOTIC

You need an antibiotic to ease, relieve, and eliminate allergic distress. This antibiotic blocks the action of allergens, cancels their irritating reactions and washes them out of your system. To use a chemicalized preparation is to introduce more "foreign offenders" into your system, and this compounds the problem. Available is a *natural* antibiotic. It is an everyday power food that corrects the *cause* of the allergy and then relieves the symptoms. This power food is *garlic.*

How Garlic Creates Natural Antibiotic Healing Benefit. This everyday power food contains two special substances: sulfides and disulfides. When eaten, these substances unite with the virus or irritating allergen in your respiratory-digestive tract, and help to inactivate them. This helps to halt their harmful effects. Reactions are soothed. Soon there is freedom from the allergic distress because of this natural antibiotic power food.

How to Use This Power Food. Chop, grate or dice one garlic clove and mix in a raw vegetable salad. Eat one garlic-containing salad in the morning, another in the afternoon, a third one in the evening. Include fresh parsley with the salad to take away any strong garlic odor. Gradually increase dosages to two chopped garlic cloves with each salad. Slowly, the antibiotic factors in this power food will cleanse your system and there will be a decline in severity of symptoms. As your allergic reactions ease, you may reduce garlic intake.

Suggestion: As a maintenance dose, plan to have one garlic bulb divided in daily salads throughout the week. This keeps your resistance high against offending allergens.

QUICK-ACTING ALLERGY-HEALING POWER FOOD TONIC

Help build a defensive wall against allergens with the help of this tasty but speedily effective allergy-healing power food tonic. It washes out offending substances. It helps you breathe better in a matter of moments. It stabilizes your metabolic rate so that formerly forbidden foods or allergy-causing edibles may now be enjoyed. It is a health-boosting tonic that will make you feel refreshed and youthfully alert.

How to Make Allergy-Healing Power Food Tonic. In one eight-ounce glass, combine six ounces of grapefruit juice, four tablespoons of very dark honey, one teaspoon of apple cider vinegar, one tablespoon of lecithin granules (from health stores or pharmacy). Blenderize for one minute, or else shake very vigorously or stir until all ingredients are blended. Now drink slowly.

Allergy-Healing Powers of Tonic. The concentrated Vitamin C of the grapefruit juice activates the iron content of the dark honey and uses this mineral to strengthen your bloodstream. This helps fight the power of allergens. This combo now sends forth the potassium from the apple cider vinegar to boost cell fluid balance and establish better electrical potential to allow stronger nerve impulse conduction so that allergen offending is reduced. Now, the nutrients combine with the high concentrates of B-complex vitamins in the lecithin to energize your neuro-respiratory system so that the irritating effect of the allergen is "knocked out" and then washed out through the bloodstream (iron-enriched from the honey) in a cleansing action. You will feel a welcome relief from allergic symptoms within 30 to 60 minutes after taking this tasty tonic.

When to Take Power Food Tonic. When you feel an allergic reaction, drink this tonic immediately. Plan to drink another full portion about four hours later. Take a third tonic still another four hours later. Now you are giving your body the working materials with which the allergens can be nullified. As a maintenance supply, drink one Power Food Tonic daily, at noontime, about an hour before a meal. The allergy-fighting ingredients will be able to work without competition from other digesting-demanding foods. This tasty *Quick-Acting Allergy-Healing Power Food Tonic* works speedily and effectively. In many situations, you should discover relief within an hour after finishing the tonic. You will look and feel much better in this short time.

HOW TO BUILD NATURAL RESISTANCE TO ALLERGIES

Just as power foods are able to correct internal disturbances so that you can resist allergies, so will improved living methods help you build natural resistance to allergies from external sources. A combination of *internal* and *external* resistance is your key to freedom from allergies.

Here's a set of suggestions offered by the American Lung Association[1] to help you build natural resistance to allergies:

1. Mattresses, pillows, and blankets should be made of allergen-free materials or enclosed in allergen-proof covers. These covers can be removed and taken on vacations and business trips.
2. Curtains should be washable and made of an allergen-free material. Washable throw rugs may also be used. Heavy drapes and carpets should not be used because they are dust collectors.
3. Your floors should be dusted and damp-mopped frequently.
4. Your closets should be kept free of unnecessary items that merely hold dust. If possible, closets should be used only for storing necessary clothing that is kept in closed garment bags.
5. Air conditioning helps filter out larger dust particles and some pollens. Some people cannot tolerate a sudden change in temperature, especially a change from warm to

---

[1]*Natural Health Bulletin*, Vol. 8, No. 16, July 31, 1978, Parker Publishing Company, West Nyack, New York 10994. Available by subscription.

cold air. So lower the temperature slowly. Don't keep your air conditioner on high.

6. Tightly fitting window filters such as those made of glass fiber or polystyrene can keep large particles ouf of the indoor air. They are effective against many pollens and spores.
7. Ninety percent of irritating particles are smaller and require an electrostatic air filter or a filter of comparable efficiency to remove them from the air. These filters are available as portable units.
8. When using any spray products, glues, paints or other chemicals around the house, cover your mouth and nose. If possible, you should also cover your eyes. Always use these products in a well-ventilated area. Using an exhaust fan in the kitchen to eliminate cooking odors is helpful.
9. Studies show that the nonsmoker is affected by smoke in the air as much as the person who smokes, so always avoid smoke-filled rooms.

With the use of power foods and an improved lifestyle,your body will be able to build natural resistance to allergens. You will then be able to help relieve and even eliminate allergic conditions.

See ASTHMA, BREATHING DIFFICULTIES, EMPHYSEMA, SINUSITIS.

ARTERIOSCLEROSIS
Power foods that melt excess fat in arteries

Arteriosclerosis is a condition characterized by clogging of the arteries with fatty deposits on the walls. If unchecked, this causes a narrowing and hardening of the arteries so that they lose their youthful flexibility. Gradually, there is a buildup of plaques in the arterial walls. This narrows the artery, often until it is blocked in one of several ways. An occlusion (a cutting off) of blood flow occurs. With this arterial wall thickening, tissues (such as smooth muscle cells) are prevented from getting oxygen while lipid (fat) deposits interfere with oxygen delivery from the blood. If this condition of excess fatty accumulation on the arterial walls is allowed to continue, it may choke off circulation and predispose to heart trouble. To protect your health and your life against this threat, you need to use easily available power foods that will help dissolve and melt away this excess fat.

THE EVERYDAY VITAMIN THAT WASHES YOUR ARTERIES

An everyday vitamin, available as a supplement (in health stores and pharmacies) and found in fresh citrus fruits, has the power to dissolve and wash away the excess fatty accumulations on your arterial walls. Vitamin C is that power food.

Natural, Quick-Acting, Effective. The artery-washing power of Vitamin C works swiftly by encouraging the synthesis in the arterial lining of substances known as *mucopolysaccharides*. These substances have a detergent-like reaction upon the accumulated arteriosclerotic plaques. They help dislodge, break up and then wash away these unhealthy deposits. Your arteries become youthfully cleansed and smoothly healthful. Vitamin C, a power food, is able to activate your body's supply of *mucopolysaccharides* and create this essential life-extending biological reaction.

How to Use This Artery-Washing Power Food. Daily, boost your intake of Vitamin C through the use of fresh citrus fruits and their juices. Try oranges, grapefruits, tangerines, lemons and limes. Other sources of Vitamin C include tomatoes, watercress, seasonal berries, cabbage, potatoes, green peppers, broccoli, cauliflower.

Power Food Supplements. Vitamin C as a supplement (available in health stores and pharmacies) reportedly is very effective in promoting an artery-washing reaction. Potencies of 1000 to 2000 milligrams daily are most effective. *Suggestion:* Crush a 1000-milligram Vitamin C tablet in a glass of orange juice. Drink one glass daily. You will nourish your metabolism with this powerhouse of Vitamin C which then works speedily to create the important artery-washing *mucopolysaccharides.*

THE GOLDEN POWER FOOD WITH DYNAMIC ARTERY-WASHING ABILITY

Ordinary gold-colored vegetable oil is a treasure trove of dynamic artery-washing ability. The secret or little-known ingredient in most free-flowing vegetable oils is known as *linoleic acid.* It is this ingredient that has the ability of softening and then speedily loosening the hard cholesterol-like deposits that cause premature aging of the arteries and the body itself.

Linoleic acid is an essential fatty acid, a substance that helps to keep your arteries more elastic and your cells and tissues in a youthfully healthy condition. Linoleic acid can create the following youth-extending benefits:

- Strengthen your capillaries and cell membranes.
- Preserve the youthfulness of your skin by regulating the water balance of your body.
- Combine with cholesterol to help transport it. Also help lower blood cholesterol levels.
- Help regular blood clotting.
- Promote growth and wound healing.
- Provide the materials from which the smooth muscle-stimulating substances, prostaglandins, are made. These substances are needed for healthful artery-washing reactions.

Power Food Sources of Linoleic Acid. Free-flowing golden oils are prime sources of this artery-washing nutrient. These include corn oil, peanut oil, safflower oil, soybean oil, sunflower oil, linseed oil, wheat germ oil, walnut oil, almond oil.

How to Use This Golden Power Food. Use in cooking wherever a fat is required. Instead of butter or margarine, use any of the golden oils listed in the preceding paragraph. Combine two tablespoons of oil with one tablespoon of lemon juice and a quarter teaspoon of honey for a delicious and artery-washing salad dressing. Add one tablespoon to any homemade soup while it is simmering. Add to stews, casseroles, and any baked or broiled main dish. To help melt away excess body fat, use four tablespoons of this golden power food daily.

The Power Food Tonic That Melts Excess Fat

Clara K. was told by her physician that she had unhealthy deposits on her arteries. Tests showed that the plaques were thickening each day. If unchecked, they threatened to close off the blood flow through her arteries. Her doctor told her to follow this simple fat-melting program:

1. Eliminate the use of hard fats in cooking. (Butter, margarine, lard were all excluded.) Trim off all visible fat from meats before cooking and before eating.
2. Each day, at noontime, Clara K. was told to drink this *Artery-Washing Power Food Tonic:* In an eight-ounce glass, combine four ounces of orange juice with four ounces of grapefruit juice. Add two teaspoons of any golden oil. Either blend, shake or stir until thoroughly combined. Flabor with a bit of honey, if desired. Drink one glass daily.

Benefits, Health Rewards. The Vitamin C in the citrus fruit juices activates the linoleic acid of the golden oil, then transports it through molecular-biological channels until it is able to help loosen and wash away accumulated arterial sludge and plaque. After five days on this simple two-step program, tests showed that Clara K.'s arteries were cleaned and healthy. Now she could be assured of a better blood circulation, a more youthful appearance, and the best reward of all—a longer lifeline!

Rebuild basic body health through the cleansing of your arteries. Wash away unwanted excess fat and you will be able to enjoy many more years of youthful health!

See Blood Enrichment, Muscular Aches, Stiffness.

ARTHRITIS
Power foods that loosen up painfully stiff joints

The miserable pain of arthritis is all too familiar to millions of people of all ages. The wrenching spasm, the gnarled muscular ache, the crippling stiffness of joints are just a few of the symptoms that are painfully endured when this ailment strikes.

The uncomfortable jolt when you try to straighten up, the agonizing pain when you try to get out of bed, a chair or in and out of a car, are signals that something has gone wrong with your metabolism. Correct this error in metabolism and you will promote a chain reaction of body healing that will help correct the distress of arthritis.

THE "WARM" POWER FOOD THAT HELPS ERASE ARTHRITIS STIFFNESS

Many arthritics instinctively seek out warm climates as a means to relieve arthritic pain. Other sources of warmth include sunshine or sunlamps. At best, sunshine and sunlamps are seasonal and limited and available only in brief situations. To provide healing warmth, special power foods are important. They will help give you year-round healing by correcting the error from within so that the disturbances is eliminated and there is hope for freedom from arthritis.

Vitamin D: How It Warms Up and Heals Arthritis. In many arthritis situations, there is a loss of bone mass and demineralization. A deficiency of Vitamin D causes progressive loss not at the inflamed region alone but throughout the entire body skeleton. This creates internal congestion and inhibits the free flow of important nutrients. If Vitamin D is severely depleted, the bones become so fragile that they break under normal everyday activities. This may cause stiffness along with a feeling of coldness so often felt by arthritics. Build resistance to this deficiency with the use of Vitamin D as a warming and healing "power food." When you take Vitamin D into your metabolic system, it activates the provitamin,

7-dehydrocholesterol, beneath the surface of your skin to release a healing oil that helps nourish your bone mass, protect against mineral loss, and create a feeling of soothing warmth. At the same time, the skeletal structure becomes strengthened so that breakage is less likely. Arthritis stiffness eases and tight joints gradually become loosened up to permit more youthful flexibility.

How to Use This Power Food. Daily, plan to take a total of 600 internal units of Vitamin D in supplement form. (Available at health stores and pharmacies.) Take 200 units with your breakfast, another 200 units at noontime and a third 200 units with your evening meal. You will gradually help rebuild your skeletal structure and correct the metabolic error involved so that you will be able to warm up your body and heal arthritis distress.

THE POWER FOOD OIL THAT LUBRICATES YOUR JOINTS

Martha B. was so troubled by worsening arthritic pain that she could scarcely hold a spoon in her hand. Auto driving was hazardous because her hands could not grip the wheel, and her feet could not manipulate the pedal as quickly as was necessary. Shoulder stiffness made her cry out with pain if she had to turn her head. Just as she felt she was becoming an invalid, a visiting nurse told her about a special power food oil. This oil was a powerhouse of natural Vitamin D that would help fortify her body and give her a storehouse of this vitamin so it could be used to promote day-after-day healing of her disturbed metabolism. Martha B. began to follow a very simple program. Each day, she would take a total of six tablespoons of any fish liver oil with her various meals. The high potency Vitamin D in the fish liver oil speedily corrected the metabolic error. Within four weeks, Martha B.'s fingers and feet were youthfully flexible. Gone was shoulder and body stiffness. Now she was as agile as a youngster!

Simple, Effective Joint-Lubricating Program. To help restore your youthful metabolism and to enjoy a pain-free lifestyle, follow this very simple but effective program, using any desired fish liver oil. You may want cod liver oil, shark liver oil, halibut liver oil, depending upon individual preference. These oils are available in health stores and pharmacies. Plan to take 600 units daily. Read labels to determine potencies. Take these 600 units in these programs:

1. Combine oil with lemon juice and a bit of honey as a salad dressing.
2. Stir two tablespoons in a glass of vegetable juice.
3. Blenderize two tablespoons in a glass of fruit juice together with some honey for a tasty and bone-nourishing potion.

Healing Benefits of Power Food. The natural Vitamin D source can help reverse the process of bone resorption (dissolving) that is a symptom of the metabolic error in arthritis. As a bone strengthener, the Vitamin D will stimulate the manufacture of osteoid matrix and its subsequent mineralization so that the entire skeleton strengthens and helps cast out the erosion of arthritis. As a natural power food, fish liver oil is a prime source of the Vitamin D that is needed to help improve the health of the arthritic and offer hope for many years of pain-free living.

THE POWER FOOD PROGRAM FOR HOLISTIC HEALING OF ARTHRITIS

Restore better body metabolism with a power food program that calls for the eating of raw or uncooked foods for a period of ten days. In so doing, you create *holistic healing* of your arthritis. This "HH" method encompasses your entire body, creating correction of disturbances, restoration of metabolic balance, improvement in your basic head-to-toe internal readjustment. The power food program for this *holistic healing* (or "HH" as it is known) calls for ten days on raw and uncooked foods.

Healing Benefit: Raw foods are prime sources of vitamins, minerals, and enzymes which are either partially or often totally destroyed in cooking. Your metabolic-skeletal structure now becomes deficient in these nutrients. The nutrients found in your bone mass (vitamins and minerals) are drawn out to be used by your deficient digestive system. This weakens your skeletal structure and the threat of arthritis becomes all too painfully real. Raw foods will nourish your metabolism and strengthen your bone mass so that the ravages of arthritis may be overcome. By devoting ten days to just a raw food program, you create an "HH" reaction that revives and regenerates your metabolic processes so that your entire body responds with better health and greater resistance to the ravages of arthritis.

Basic "HH" Raw Food Arthritis-Healing Program

- *Breakfast:* Seasonal fruit compote, either sliced, diced or chopped, seasoned with a dusting of cinnamon. Assorted seeds, nuts. Soaked raw oatmeal in milk. Citrus fruit platter. Fruit or vegetable juice.
- *Mid-Morning:* Platter of sun-dried fruits sprinkled with wheat germ and bran flakes. Herb tea with honey and lemon juice.
- *Luncheon:* Raw vegetable salad with dressing made of two tablespoons of cod liver oil, two tablespoons apple cider vinegar, and desired herbs. Fresh fruit salad, with sun-dried raisins. Herb tea with honey and lemon juice or any desired coffee substitute.
- *Mid-Afternoon:* Vegetable juice cocktail.
- *Dinner:* Fruit puree flavored with honey or maple syrup. Chopped nuts and seeds on lettuce leaves with tomato wedges. Apple wedges sprinkled with cinnamon. Herb tea with honey and lemon juice.
- *Before Bedtime:* Vegetable juice cocktail.

Suggestions for "HH" Program: For ten days, vary your selection of any currently available fruits and vegetables. You can enjoy new taste thrills each day on this program with different seasonal foods. Chew all raw foods well to release important enzymes that will be able to metabolize the swallowed foods so that healing nutrients will be taken up by your bloodstream and carried to your ailing skeletal structure. This helps correct the metabolic error that is to blame for your arthritis distress. Whenever you eat, do so calmly. Be of good cheer. This helps improve enzymatic digestion and metabolic correction.

Nature-created substances in these raw foods help balance

your metabolism, and this is the key to freedom from arthritis. These are power foods that energize your sluggish metabolism to promote whole body or *holistic healing.*

After your ten-day program, ease into cooked foods. But plan to eat raw foods more frequently as a maintenance program for better health. Raw foods are the power foods that will help you loosen up your tight or congested joints and open an avenue for escape from arthritis.

Help your body heal itself with the use of power foods!

See Bone Ailments, Bursitis, Gout, Muscular Aches, Stiffness.

ASTHMA
Power foods that refresh your lungs

Asthma is a condition characterized by coughing, wheezing and difficult breathing. It may be caused by an allergen, either inhaled or swallowed. The condition may be made worse at times by emotional reactions to strain. Asthma may begin at any age, often in the form of hay fever. If neglected, it tends to recur and may become chronic. To help build resistance to asthmatic offenders, follow the same lung-strengthening program as recommended[1] for hay fever:

1. Do not drink alcohol. It dilates your blood vessels and may precipitate an attack.
2. Try not to have any arguments or become involved in stressful situations. Emotional tension often sets off asthmatic attacks.
3. Do not overexert yourself and become fatigued. Do not make drastic changes from one temperature to another. For example, you should not go from a cool indoors to a hot outdoors without waiting in a neutral area to allow your body to adjust to the change.

---

[1]*Natural Health Bulletin,* June 5, 1978, Volume 8, No. 12, Parker Publishing Company, West Nyack, New York 10994. Available by subscription.

4. Do not eat or drink anything that is icy cold or extremely hot. Do not eat heavily spiced foods or beverages.
5. Give up smoking. It chokes the respiratory organs and can trigger off an attack.
6. Do not swim in a chlorinated pool. If you're swimming in an ocean or lake, do not suddenly plunge into the cold water. Ease yourself in slowly.
7. Listen to local weather forecasts or call your local health department for the daily ragweed pollen count. If the count is high, do not open windows. Stay indoors in an air-conditioned environment as much as possible. Take care that your room does not become too chilly. A lung-soothing temperature is about 75°F.
8. Avoid using powdered soaps and insecticides.
9. Do not cut flowers or do any gardening or household painting. These activities may irritate the respiratory tract and cause an attack.
10. Do not go for a ride in the country unless you know the area is reasonably free of pollen. Otherwise, you may suffer an attack which may linger for hours.

By pampering your respiratory tract, you will strengthen your body so it can make more beneficial use of power foods that will act as natural asthma healers.

THE POWER FOOD THAT OPENS "LOCKED" LUNGS

Any citrus fruit is a powerhouse of Vitamin C which is needed to rebuild and repair the fragile tissues of the bronchial system housing the lungs. By boosting your daily intake of fresh oranges and grapefruit and tangerines, you will be nourishing your lungs with healing Vitamin C. When the cells and tissues of your lungs are rebuilt with Vitamin C, they open up to let you breathe healthfully with freedom from asthmatic choking.

How Fruits Opened "Locked" Lungs in Three Days. As a computer systems analyst, Morton J. was required to make daily reports to his supervisors about work in progress. Morton J. was frequently embarrassed by severe outbreaks of asthmatic choking and gasping for precious air. He made a poor impression because of these sudden attacks. His job was in jeopardy.

Morton J. tried chemical medications but they gave him such allergic side effects that his symptoms worsened. Soon he began to look aged and haggard. The constant choking and sputtering drained away his health and vitality.

A company nurse-nutritionist put him on a special power food program that emphasized Vitamin C. After just three days on this power food program, his asthmatic symptoms subsided. Now he could breathe with youthful health. The power food program consisting of citrus fruits had opened his "locked" lungs in three days. Life became joyful again!

Citrus Power Foods for Lung Refreshment. A lung-healing program calls for eating fresh citrus fruits daily. These include oranges, grapefruit, tangerines. A platter consisting of citrus fruit on a bed of lettuce leaves and tomato wedges with a few slices of cucumber will give you a powerhouse of lung-healing Vitamin C. To rebuild your breathing system and resist the irritants that cause asthmatic attack, plan to eat at least two ample citrus fruit salads daily.

Healing Power of Citrus Power Foods. Citrus fruits are prime sources of Vitamin C which is needed to rebuild the capillaries of your lungs. Capillaries are small blood vessels that crisscross the tissues of your bronchial-breathing components. Through the walls of these capillaries, food and oxygen are transported to nourish the lungs so they will resist offenders that could trigger off an asthmatic attack. Vitamin C is the dynamic power food that assists in the formation of collagen (connective tissue) which strengthens the integrity and stability of your lung and breathing organ tissues. This creates a protective wall-like enclosure surrounding your lungs so that irritants will not be able to penetrate. Breathing becomes refreshingly youthful and healthy again. Nourish your lungs with an abundant supply of Vitamin C through daily intake of fresh citrus fruits.

Citrus Fruit Juices: Right Vs. Wrong Way to Use Them. As lung-refreshing power foods, citrus fruit juices are superior in helping you resist and overcome asthmatic difficulties. But there is a right and a wrong way to use them. The *right* way is to drink a glass of pure orange juice (freshly prepared or from a bottled source if the label says it is pure) only if it is comfortably cool—not ice-chilled. The *wrong* way is to drink it when it is icy cold or frozen cold. Frigid citrus fruit juice (or any other juice) will cause narrowing and constriction of the delicate tubules of your breathing components. This will trigger off an asthmatic attack. For soothing and healing comfort, juices should be cool but *not* icy cold!

Power Food Asthma-Healing Tonics. In the morning, drink a glass of orange juice; mid-morning, a glass of grapefruit juice; lunchtime, a combination of orange and grapefruit juice; mid-afternoon, a glass of tangerine juice; dinnertime, a combination of orange-grapefruit-tangerine juice. Plan to drink at least one quart of these citrus juices daily, in any desired combination. They will give your lungs a rich supply of cell-building Vitamin C, the power food that helps promote healing of asthma.

THE POWER FOOD HERB THAT DISSOLVES ASTHMATIC MUCUS

Dissolve the choking mucus that makes breathing so distressful with a simple everyday power food herb. It is *fenugreek*. Available in seed form in almost all health stores and pharmacies, this herb contains natural dehydrating properties that will dissolve accumulated mucus from the nasal and respiratory passages. Breathing now becomes much easier and youthfully comfortable.

Power Food Fenugreek Tea. Add one teaspoon of fenugreek seeds to one cup of freshly boiled water. Let it steep five minutes. Add a bit of lemon juice and honey for flavoring. Plan to drink three to five cups of this power food daily. It will help dissolve mucus, and clear up your choked and stuffed breathing components. Asthmatic attacks will gradually be less severe as they fade away.

Power Food Syrup. Folklorists suggest this asthma-healing, lung-strengthening power food syrup. Put thinly sliced onions on a dish. Cover each slice with honey. Cover with an inverted plate. Let remain overnight. Next morning, you will have syrup on the plate.

Discard the onion slices. Take one teaspoon of this power food syrup in the morning, a second teaspoon at bedtime. The syrup is supercharged with potassium from the volatile onion and soothing honey, along with other essential minerals, vitamins and enzymes. This combination helps to soothe asthmatic distress and improve the breathing power of the lungs, and helps you meet the responsibilities of the day without coughing spasms. It helps you sleep better, too. It is the key to better breathing, better health and longer life, too.

Open up new air channels, refresh your lungs, rebuild your bronchial tubes and enjoy life with these wonder foods.

See Allergies, Breathing Difficulties, Emphysema, Smoking.

BACKACHE
Power foods that help to limber up painful muscles

Muscle malnutrition is a major cause of many back disorders. You can correct this deficiency and ease distressful pain by nourishing the cells, tissues and components of your musculoskeletal system (muscles, bones, joints that comprise over 60% of the total body mass).

Adequate nutrition will soothe and comfort gnarled, twisted and hurtful muscles. By using basic back-pampering programs as well as simple home muscle-energizers, you should be able to limber up your painful muscles and enjoy freedom from back distress.

THE POWER FOOD THAT NOURISHES BACK MUSCLES AND RELIEVES PAIN

A simple nutrient, available as a supplement in health stores or pharmacies, is able to nourish your back muscles, heal and relieve pain, often in a short time. It provided swift healing for a physician as well as for many of his patients. According to C. James Greenwood, Jr., M.D., clinical professor of neurosurgery at Baylor College of Medicine in Houston, Texas, Vitamin C, the simple nutrient, works quickly to help heal backache and reduce pain for many back disorders.

Relieves Soreness. Says Dr. Greenwood,[1] "Vitamin C's most dramatic immediate effect is to prevent and relieve soreness resulting from unusual exercise, such as a hunting trip, wading through marshes or sailing. It is also effective in relieving most generalized backaches."

How Power Food Works to Heal Back Pain. Vitamin C is a building material needed to mobilize and construct collagen, a protein substance responsible for holding the body together, i.e., supporting tendons, bone, cartilage, involved in back support. Neurosurgeon Greenwood recognizes that this Vitamin C acts as a power food to nourish the starved components of the back and ease pain as well as protect against recurring distress.

Power Food Program. Take 1500 milligrams of Vitamin C a day ahead of any anticipated heavy physical exertion. This fortifies your musculoskeletal system and strengthens your back muscles so there is greater resistance to ache. Dr. Greenwood reports that when his patients and his colleagues follow this simple power food program, they all enjoy relief from muscle soreness.

Power Food Protects Against Backache. Troubled with back pain himself, Dr. Greenwood reports taking 100 milligrams of Vitamin C three times daily for four months. "I could then exercise without any difficulty. When I discontinued the Vitamin C program, my back pain returned." So it was clear that this power food offered hope for freedom of back distress. Dr. Greenwood prescribed Vitamin C to more than 500 of his patients who had back trouble, and reports "gratifying relief as long as they continue with Vitamin C."

Back-Nourishing Program. Dr. Greenwood recommends taking 1500 milligrams of Vitamin C a day, divided into portions of 500 milligrams with each meal. This helps nourish the back's skeletal system and offers protection against health-draining bachaches and

---

[1]*Medical Annals of the District of Columbia*, Washington, D.C., June, 1964.

pains. Power food healing is one part of the program to enjoy a healthy and resilient back. "Adequate nutrition, including optimum Vitamin C and *daily exercise* will eliminate many back pains, strains and disk ruptures," concludes Dr. Greenwood.

Do the following exercises twice a day

(each one three times)

These exercises are designed to strengthen the muscles of your lower back and abdomen and thus help prevent a recurrence of your low-back problem. You should not do them when you are actually in pain. Always follow your doctor's instructions.

Knee Hug

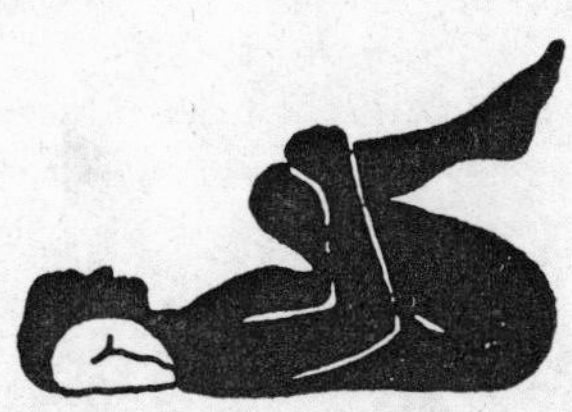

1. Lie on back, pillow under head, arms at side. Inhale.
2. Slowly raise knees to chest.
3. Bring up hands and clasp knees as tightly as you can. Exhale.
4. Hold for count of 10. Relax.

Back Flattener

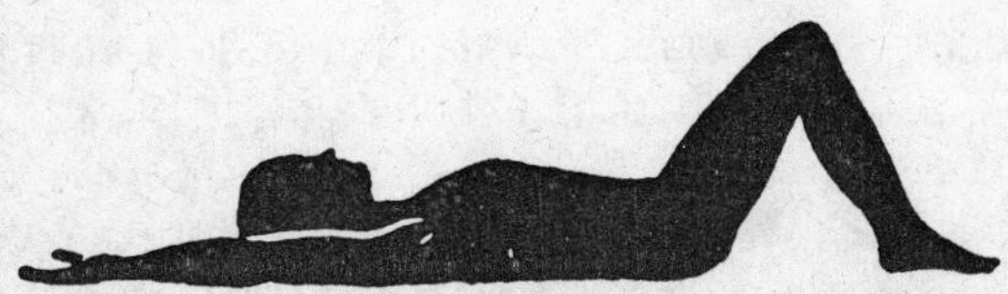

1. Lie on back, knees raised, feet on floor, hands over head. Relax.
2. Tighten stomach and buttocks muscles at same time to flatten back against floor.
3. Hold for a count of 10. Relax.

Stomach Firmer

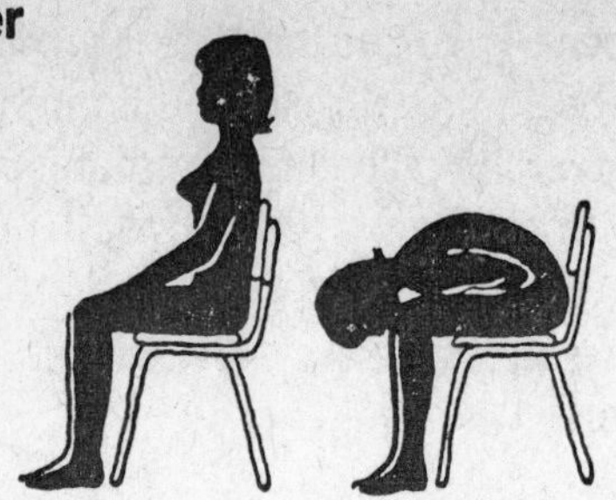

1. Sit on hard chair, arms folded loosely in lap.
2. Let head drop forward until it is between knees.
3. Tighten abdominal muscles and hold.
4. Slowly pull your body to a sitting position. Relax.

Posture Check

(to help you stand and walk correctly)

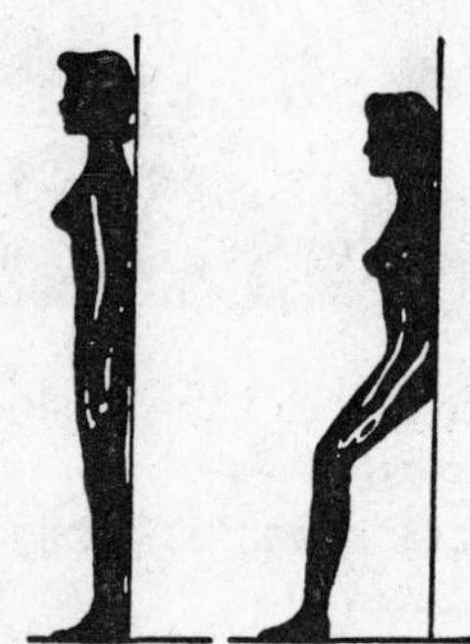

1. Stand with back to wall. Press heels, rump, shoulders, and head against wall. If you feel any space between small of back and wall, your back is arched too much.
2. Move feet forward and bend knees so that your back slides a few inches down wall. Now, tighten abdominal and buttocks muscles so you can flatten lower back against wall.
3. Hold this position and "walk" your feet back so that you slide up wall.
4. Standing straight, walk away from wall and around the room.
5. Return to wall and back up to it to make sure you've kept proper posture.

BACKACHE-HEALING POWER FOOD ELIXIR

A combination of important nutrients in an easy-to-make *Backache-Healing Power Food Elixir* will help nourish the various muscle-bone components of your back. This eases distress and will help promote healing of your back. Here is how to make and take this back-healing beverage:

How to Make: In one eight-ounce glass, pour six ounces of skim milk, two tablespoons non-fat dry milk powder, one tablespoon cod liver oil, one tablespoon honey, four tablespoons orange juice. Blenderize for one minute or else stir or shake vigorously until all ingredients are combined.

How to Take: Drink one glass of this back-healing elixir in the morning. Drink a second glass at noontime. Drink a third glass in the evening.

Heals Swiftly. Anna May E. was constantly troubled with painful back spasms. Bending over to vacuum brought such sharp knife-like pain that she would cry out in anguish. She had to stop housework and rest until the throbbing subsided. Even afterward, she felt warning spasms and had to work slowly, if at all. An osteopathic physician recommended that she try the *Backache-Healing Power Food Elixir*, three times daily. It was miraculous. Within two days, her back had limbered up. Gone were aches. Vanished were pains. Now she felt more youthful as she could work with vitality and energy.

Benefits of Elixir: The power healing benefits in the elixir consist of the unique combination of calcium, Vitamin C and Vitamin D. When swallowed, the calcium becomes energized by the Vitamin C. It is then propelled by Vitamin D through the back's musculoskeletal system. Healing now takes place. The milk calcium, the fruit juice Vitamin C and the oil Vitamin D *must be present in this combination* for power food healing. The calcium, in particular, now becomes stored inside the ends of bones in long, needlelike crystals called *trabeculae*. Here, the calcium is measured out through the Vitamin C plus D influence to nourish your important structural bones to help heal and protect against back distress.

HOW TO BE GOOD TO YOUR BACK FOR FREEDOM FROM ACHES AND PAINS

Protect yourself against back distress with these suggestions:

Sitting Advice:

1. At home or work, sit in a straight chair with a firm back.
2. Sit so that your knees are higher than your hips. To do this you may need a small footstool.
3. Avoid sitting in swivel chairs and chairs on rollers.
4. Do not sit in overstuffed chairs or sofas.
5. Never sit in the same position for prolonged periods. Get up and move around.

Driving Advice:

6. Push the front seat of your car forward so your knees will be higher than your hips. This will reduce the strain on back and shoulder muscles.
7. Always fasten safety belt and shoulder harness.
8. A headrest may be helpful.

Standing and Walking Advice:

9. Don't stand in the same position for longer than a few minutes. Shift from one foot to the other.
10. When standing don't lean back and support your body with your hands. Keep hands in front of your body and lean forward slightly.
11. When turning to walk from a standing position, move your feet first and then your body, for better balance.
12. Open doors wide enough to walk through comfortably.
13. Carefully judge the height of curbs before stepping up or down.
14. Women should change to low heels frequently.

Bed Rest Advice:

15. If your doctor prescribes *absolute* bed rest, stay in bed. Raising your body or twisting and turning can put a severe strain on your back.

16. When lying flat on your back, it may help to put pillows under your knees (unless your physician recommends otherwise).
17. When sleeping, lie on your side and draw one or both knees up toward your chin.
18. When lying in bed, don't extend your arms above your head. Relax them at your side.
19. Do not sleep on your stomach.
20. Sleep on a flat, firm mattress.
21. A bed board (½ inch to ¾ inch thick) placed between your mattress and box springs is an excellent support for your back.

Lifting Advice:

22. When lifting, let your legs do the work, not your back. This applies even if you're picking up a scrap of paper.
23. Squat directly in front of the object you plan to lift, keeping it close to your body. Then slowly rise to a standing position.
24. Never lift with your legs straight.
25. Don't lift from a bending forward position.
26. Don't lift heavy objects from car trunks.
27. Don't reach over furniture to open and close windows.
28. When two or more persons plan to lift something, they should decide in advance what each is going to do, so one of them doesn't get caught with a sudden, unexpected load.

Yard Work Advice:

29. A little exercise every day is far better than a whole lot on the weekend.
30. Before working in your yard or garden, be sure to warm up.
31. To warm up, swing the tool you plan to use (rake, hoe, axe, mattock, etc.) lazily back and forth around your head and shoulders in different positions, gradually working up to the full range of motion and effort needed to do the job.

Remember that athletes always warm up before taking vigorous exercise.

32. Wear protective clothing to keep your perspiring body from getting chilled, except on very warm days. Remember that a baseball pitcher always puts on a warm-up jacket as soon as he leaves the mound.
33. The weekend golfer, fisherman or tennis player should take along extra clothing to avoid getting chilled late in the day.
34. Don't go into an air-conditioned building while you're perspiring.

Miscellaneous Advice:

35. Don't make up beds or run the vacuum cleaner if your back is acting up.
36. A prolonged, comfortably hot bath can be relaxing for a strained back. Be sure the water isn't too hot.
37. Your doctor may recommend some simple exercises to help strengthen the low-back and stomach muscles. Always follow his directions.
38. Avoid overweight.

Be good to your back through improved nutrition, the healing of power foods and the guidelines described above. By so doing, your back will be youthfully good to you, too!

See ARTHRITIS, BURSITIS, MUSCULAR ACHES, SPINAL COLUMN, STIFFNESS.

BLADDER
Power foods that soothe and control bladder functions

The bladder is the membranous sac that collects and stores urine from the kidneys. It is located in the front part of the pelvic cavity. It is a collapsible, balloonlike sac composed of smooth muscle and lined with a smooth membrane. Its size and shape are determined by the amount of urine it contains. The bladder's outlet is protected by a strong sphincter muscle which is firmly contracted except during voiding. As urine collects in the bladder, the sensory nerves in its walls become stimulated. These nerve impulses are transmitted by way of the spinal cord to the brain. When the sphincter muscle relaxes, then voiding is possible. This is partly a reflex and partly a learned reaction.

Should the mucous membrane lining the bladder become unhealthfully irritated or inflamed, the nerve bulbs will signal an almost constant urge to void, despite the amount of fluid that is actually present. This represents a nutritional disturbance in the membranous sac and its neuromuscular components.

An inadequate amount of urine voided may cause precipitation of solids and the risk of bladder stone formation. An excess amount of urine voided may be symptomatic of tense bladder muscles which compel frequent bathroom trips even though the bladder is far from being full. These extremes are nature's warning signals that corrective nutritional methods need to be followed to improve the health of the bladder and the rest of the body.

Acid-Plus Urine = Healthy Bladder. Slightly acidic urine indicates a healthy bladder. The benefit here is that when you use power foods and power juices to increase the acid of your urine, there is greater protection against infection and stone formation. If there is a deficiency in acid-forming power foods and power juices, minerals that are filtered out of the blood for excretion can become solid, forming into stones in the urinary tract. But with acidic urine, the minerals can be dissolved and are then washed out of the system. To protect against the problem of stone formation, use power foods and power juices to create acid-plus urine, the key to a healthy bladder.

THE POWER JUICE THAT KEEPS YOUR BLADDER YOUTHFULLY HEALTHY

Cranberry juice has a tart flavor because the fruit is more acid than alkaline in growth as well as in digestion. Cranberry juice is a power food that will help nourish the membranes and muscles of the bladder and thereby help acidify the urine so that it is able to keep dissolved minerals in a solution to be passed off. Otherwise, these minerals may cling together and form crystal-like stones that become lodged in the bladder. Cranberry juice is a prime source of potassium, a mineral that will help bladder muscles to contract and also help to maintain bladder cell fluid balance.

Power Juice Bladder-Healing Program. Plan to drink two glasses of cranberry juice daily. Drink one glass at noontime; drink a second glass at dinnertime. The nutrients in this power juice will help stimulate a healthy release of acid so that urine will be youthfully tart, dissolving wastes and then washing them out of your system. Your bladder will also benefit from the Vitamin C content in the cranberry juice. The vitamin will build stronger cells and blood vessels of the bladder, thereby giving it (and your body) better health and longer life.

FOLK REMEDIES TO REVIVE-REGENERATE-REJUVENATE YOUR BLADDER

If you are troubled by having to get up at night for frequent voiding, or if your problem is too infrequent voiding, then you need to revive-regenerate-rejuvenate your bladder with folk remedies that act swiftly as power foods.

New England Bladder-Rejuvenating Power Food. Create a youthful acid-ackaline urine balance (with emphasis on acid) with the use of apple cider vinegar, as do folks in New England. Just stir two tablespoons of this high-potassium and naturally acid vinegar into a glass of water. Add one tablespoon of honey for taste. Blenderize a moment or stir until combined. Now sip slowly. Just one glass a day (divided into two portions, if desired) will help nourish your bladder and also slightly acidify your urine so that wastes can be liquified and washed out of your body. It is a tangy power food that helps keep your bladder (and body) young!

Vitamin C: Bladder-Healing Power Food. In several reports,[1] physicians were able to improve and heal the bladder with the use of an everyday power food—Vitamin C.

A team of physicians gave patients doses of Vitamin C amounting to 4000 milligrams daily. The patients had improved bladder health and desired urine acidity.

[1]*Journal of the American Medical Association,* Chicago, Illinois, April 21, 1975. *N. Y. State Journal of Medicine*, Buffalo, N.Y., December 15, 1971.

A group of men were troubled with urethritis (irritation of the urethra, the canal that conveys urine from the bladder neck to the outside). The problem was traced to the accumulation of phosphatic crystals. Doctors gave each man 3000 milligrams of Vitamin C each day for just four days. Results? This power food helped heal the condition and symptoms vanished.

Healing Power. The irritating phosphatic crystals had formed in the urine which was low in acid. Vitamin C as a power food was able to create an acid-plus condition in the urine and this broke down the crystals so they could be washed out of the system. At the same time, the simple daily dosage of this power food also revived and regenerated the health of the bladder.

Bean Pod Juice for Bladder Regeneration. Folk healers suggest this remedy for bladder regeneration and better body health: boil two ounces of kidney bean pods (not the beans) in four quarts of water for four hours. Strain and cool. Plan to drink one glass of this bean pod juice every four hours. It is said that this folk healer helps create a normal acid-alkaline urine and also soothes and even eliminates pain. It also helps to stimulate voiding as dissolved crystals are washed out of the system.

Be good to your bladder by pampering it with nutritious foods. Avoid foods or beverages that are too hot or too cold. These shock your bladder and it reacts violently. Use natural herbs and spices for flavoring instead of volatile salt and pepper. Your bladder will serve you for a longer and healthier lifespan.

See Colitis, Constipation, Cramps, Diarrhea, Digestive Ddisturbances, Kidneys, Liver, Urinary Problems.

BLOOD ENRICHMENT
Power foods that nourish blood cells

A rich, healthy bloodstream is your river of life. Your body will resist ailments and enjoy greater health and much longer youthful life when it is washed and nourished with an alert and invigorated bloodstream.

Your circulatory system is responsible for the continuous delivery of oxygenated blood and its nutrients to all body cells and tissues, the exchange for waste products of metabolism, and transportation of wastes to points of elimination. Without a supply of oxygenated and nutrient-carrying blood, body cells and tissues as well as vital organs start to deteriorate and the aging process is underway. A nutrient-carrying bloodstream helps you fight infections, and plays a defensive role against aging through the filtering action of special lymph glands (channels that remove impurities and harmful microbes). Your bloodstream also creates and adds defensive elements such as antibodies to your system to help resist age-causing ailments.

Bloodstream: Body Conveyor System. Your blood conveys oxygen from your lungs to your cells. Then it conveys carbon dioxide from your tissues back to your lungs where it will be cast out with your exhalation. Your blood picks up digestive-intestinal nutrients which are transported through your liver to your body cells and tissues. This conveyor system then takes waste substances from your cells and transports them to your organs of elimination. A healthy bloodstream will convey cell-tissue-organ nutrients to all parts of your body from head to toe. It is the source of perpetual and extended youthful health.

One-Minute Do-It-Yourself Blood Health Test. To determine if your bloodstream is sluggish, try this simple test. It takes just one minute. Press your fingertips very firmly against any hard surface (desk, table top, windowsill, shelf) for just 45 seconds. Are your fingernails very red or very pink? If so, it indicates that you do have a good and active bloodstream. If your fingernails remained pale as you pressed your fingers down on the surface, it suggests you may have a sluggish bloodstream in need of power food nourishment for greater activity. *Caution:* A sluggish bloodstream means it may have a tendency to form clots and this could be a health risk! You can find this out within one minute by following this test.

THE EVERYDAY POWER FOOD THAT NOURISHES YOUR BLOOD CELLS

Polyunsaturated vegetable oil is a highly concentrated source of Vitamin E, a nutrient that is needed to nourish and invigorate the vigor and youthful health of your blood cells.

Wheat germ oil, safflower seed oil, corn oil, peanut oil, sesame seed oil, sunflower seed oil are all prime sources of Vitamin E. This power food nutrient is able to increase the amount of oxygen for your body cells, tissues and organs. It also prevents the oxidation of fatty acids in the blood so that your cells become better nourished and more vigorous in protecting you from ill health.

Blood Cell Feeding Program. Daily, add four tablespoons of any of the aforementioned power food oils to your raw vegetable salad. Combine with some apple cider vinegar and lemon juice for a tasty and blood-feeding salad dressing. You will be giving your blood cells the much-needed Vitamin E to help give you better health and longer life.

COPPER: THE POWER FOOD THAT INVIGORATES YOUR RED BLOOD CELLS

As a power food, copper is essential to form hemoglobin, the red coloring matter of your blood. It transports nutrient-bearing oxygen to all parts of your body. Copper is used to invigorate your brain, rejuvenate your liver cells, become involved in skin pigment formation. Copper functions in the synthesis of red blood cells and the oxidation systems of your body. It is needed for repair and regeneration of body cells and tissues. Your bloodstream "drinks" copper which gives it a source of youthful vigor that is then shared with your body organs so that you will respond with better health.

Cell-Feeding Copper Tonic. In one large glass of citrus fruit juice, add two tablespoons of brewer's yeast, one tablespoon of lecithin, and a quarter-teaspoon of honey. Blenderize or stir until all items are assimilated. Drink just one glass of this *Cell-Feeding Copper Tonic* daily to give your red blood cells a powerhouse of much-needed copper. Almost immediately, the mineral is used to rebuild the red cells of your bloodstream so they can transport needed nutrients and oxygen to all body parts. You will feel yourself glow with youthful vitality in a little while, thanks to the power in this tonic.

The enzymes and Vitamin C in the fruit juice activate the copper in both the brewer's yeast and lecithin and stimulate the mineral so it is more speedily and effectively assimilated. Both brewer's yeast and lecithin are grain products available in most health stores and pharmacies. Use them for greater blood and body health.

POWER FOODS THAT BUILD IMMUNITY TO DISORDERS

Build immunity and freedom from disorders with a healthy and invigorated lymph system. The purpose of lymph (straw colored portion of your blood) is to serve as a sentry in your immunologic system of defense against infection and harmful microbes. The lymph acts as a filter by protecting your bloodstream from potentially harmful invaders. Nourish your lymph with these power foods:

Immunity Building Power Food. Prepare a platter of raw citrus fruits (orange wedges, grapefruit wedges, sprinkled with lemon juice). Break open a capsule of 500 milligrams of Vitamin C. Sprinkle over salad. Eat one such salad daily. You will be sending a source of powerful Vitamin C to your lymph system, which will use it to strengthen cells and tissues to act as barriers against harmful infectious agents.

Blood-Building Fruits. Sun-dried apricots, prunes, raisins, dates, figs are powerhouses of iron and copper as well as Vitamins A and C which are able to generate a magnetic blood current and an electromagnetic induction current in the circulatory system so that there is an increase in the quantity and quality of lymph and white blood cells needed to build resistance to infections. Eat these fruits daily to nourish your blood circulation.

Infection-Fighting Natural Sweet. Called blackstrap molasses (available in health stores and many supermarkets), it is the product of the last extraction of the sugar cane. It is a powerhouse of highly concentrated minerals, especially copper and iron. These nutrients found in this natural sweet help form hemoglobin and also myoglobin, a substance that stores oxygen in your cells and tissues, gives you greater stamina, and promotes an increase in much-needed lymph so that infection is both resisted and controlled and eventually eliminated through metabolic processes. Use two teaspoons of molasses for flavoring in herb tea. Use it as a healthy sugar or refined sweet substitute. You will enjoy its taste. At the same time, your blood will become richer and you will enjoy better health and a longer lifespan.

Your river of life will flow with vigor and strength when properly nourished through the stimulation of healthy and life-extending power foods.

See CIRCULATION, IRON.

BLOOD PRESSURE (HIGH AND LOW)
Power foods that balance levels

Unbalanced blood pressure (too high or too low) is a time bomb ticking away in your body. When it goes off, your health and your very life are put in jeopardy. A problem with unbalanced blood pressure is that it reveals few if any symptoms, which is why it is called a "sneaky" condition.

High Blood Pressure. Also known as hypertension, it is a condition in which there is a persistently elevated blood pressure. (Blood pressure refers to the amount of pressure exerted in the bloodstream as it passes through the arteries.) Everyone needs blood pressure to move blood through the circulatory system. This pressure varies; it goes up and down within a limited range. When it goes up and stays up, it is called high blood pressure. This places the heart and arteries under unhealthy strain. Symptoms are almost non-existent. It can be detected through a doctor's blood pressure test. Otherwise, it may go unnoticed and continue "ticking" until a stroke, blood clot, heart attack or kidney malfunction results and then the condition is exposed!

Low Blood Pressure. Also known as hypotension, it is a condition which is symptomatic of poor nutrition. There may be disorders such as low blood sugar, low basal metabolism, below-normal temperature, anemia and a sluggish thyroid gland. Hypotensive folks are less energetic because of this glandular slowdown. There may be some symptoms such as vertigo (dizziness) and a light-headed feeling when sitting up after being in bed for a long time, or even when standing up after having sat for a while. A problem here is that when you want to stand up or make any posture change, your circulation must instantly send a supply of blood to your brain cells to effect this change. But in hypotension there is a sluggish blood pressure. This causes a sluggish transportation system. It takes longer for blood to go to your brain cells. Signals to change posture are slow moving. If this condition is neglected, the body systems grow weaker and weaker until the entire organism becomes inactive.

Let us see how everyday power foods can help balance your blood pressure and add years of good health to a longer lifespan.

POWER FOOD PROGRAM TO BALANCE HIGH BLOOD PRESSURE

1. **Eliminate Salt in All Forms.** Salt or sodium chloride, whether used at the table, in cooking or in packaged-processed foods, should be eliminated. Salt whips up glandular action to release substances that constrict the passageways of the small arteries. This leads to high blood pressure. *Power Food Suggestions:* Flavorful herbs and spices that are salt-and sodium chloride-free should be used as a replacement. Use lemon or lime juice as a tart flavoring. Available in health stores and supermarkets, these power food replacements are gentle to your system and will help control blood pressure.

2. **Eliminate Sugar in All Forms.** Refined sugar used at the table, in cooking or in packaged-processed foods should also be eliminated. Sugar causes glandular disturbance, overstimulates the isles of Langerhans (insulin-producing cells in the pancreas), and this creates erratic and nervous temperament that induces high blood pressure. *Power Food Suggestions:* Honey, blackstrap molasses, maple syrup, berry juices and sweet herbs and spices are good sugar replacements. They contain nutrients that soothe your blood pressure while satisfying your desire for a sweet taste.

3. **Eliminate Caffeine in All Forms.** This crystallizable, slightly bitter, stimulating alkaloid found in the leaves and berries of tne coffee plant is used in coffee, cola drinks and many other soft drinks, in some confections such as chocolates and also in some

commercial teas. The caffeine upsets the balance of the nervous system, especially the higher centers, and triggers off a speedier respiratory rate. Caffeine will also cause a vaso-dilatation of the peripheral blood vessels, causing erratic blood pressure behavior. Tachycardia (increased heartbeat) and extra systoles (irregular heart function) are frequent. Caffeine should be eliminated for the health of your body and blood pressure balance. *Power Food Suggestions:* Use caffeine-free beverages (read the labels) and herbal teas as well as any of the coffee substitutes (such as Postum) available in health stores and almost all supermarkets. To quench your thirst, try fruit and vegetable juices which contain vitamins and minerals that will soothe your nervous system and relax your blood pressure.

POWER FOODS THAT SOOTHE YOUR BLOOD PRESSURE

Soothe and regulate your blood pressure by nourishing your metabolism with these power foods. They are so called because they create a form of biological power to healthfully influence the rate of force involved in pushing blood through your system. By eating (and enjoying) these power foods, your body receives nutrients required to create a healthy force of blood pressure.

- *Whole Grains:* Oats, millet, bran, wheat germ, brown rice, unpearled barley or bulgur wheat are prime sources of *natural* carbohydrates which energize your system and soothe your nerves so that your pressure becomes more stabilized.
- *Almonds:* A good source of plant protein. High in many amino acids that strengthen your vascular walls and help you maintain better blood force balance.
- *Apples and Apple Juice:* A prime source of malic acid, a nutrient that helps relax your body and thereby control erratic blood pressure.
- *Berries and Berry Juice:* Natural fruit juices are powerhouses of Vitamin C which is needed to strengthen the cells and tissues of the arteries and thereby help contain the throbbing force so it does not become unhealthfully overactive.

- *Pineapple:* Contains *bromelain*, an enzyme that creates healing and repair of weakened arterial walls so that the force of blood is eased and controlled. Also helps improve digestive metabolism. When internal congestion is relieved through better assimilation, the entire body responds with more youthful health.
- *Salt-Free, Skim-Milk Products:* Good sources of calcium, a soothing mineral that helps control the circumstances contributing to an elevated blood pressure. Select products (milk, cheeses, yogurt) that are salt-free or low-salt. Read labels. These are currently available in many health stores and supermarkets. They soothe and relax the body and this helps level off blood pressure.

Plan to eat these power foods regularly, along with your salt-free, sugar-free, caffeine-free pressure-balancing program.

POWER FOOD PROGRAM TO BALANCE TOO-LOW BLOOD PRESSURE

Low blood pressure, or hypotension, may be gently and healthfully balanced by increasing intake of thiamine (B_1), a vitamin that reportedly helps invigorate the sluggish system. Another power food is that of protein, which helps improve general health but specifically alerts sluggish responses to a more youthful activity. This helps improve blood pressure force to a healthful level. Here is a two-step power food program to relieve low blood pressure.

1. Brewer's Yeast for Better Pressure Balance. The dried pulverized cells of the yeast plant, this power food is a highly concentrated source of most known nutrients, especially thiamine. This nutrient is used to nourish your vascular cells and promote a better circulation as well as invigoration of your nervous system. This improves your blood pressure so it can serve you healthfully.

Power Food Potion: Blenderize one tablespoon of brewer's yeast in a glass of tomato juice. Drink three glasses daily. The powerhouse of thiamine combines with other nutrients to alert and activate your sluggish system so you respond with a healthier blood pressure level.

2. **Protein Creates Youthfully Healthy Blood Pressure.** If you lack first class protein, you may suffer from an unhealthy drop in blood pressure. Since blood vessels are largely made up of protein, a deficiency causes wasting and flabbiness which can create havoc with blood pressure. You need a daily supply of first-class protein for vascular nutrition and pressure balancing.

Power Food Potion: In a glass of skim milk, add one tablespoon of non-fat dry milk powder, one tablespoon of unflavored gelatin, one tablespoon of lecithin, one tablespoon honey or blackstrap molasses. Blenderize one minute. Drink three glasses daily. You will send a tremendous powerhouse of first class protein, energized by the *natural* sugars in the sweeteners, to strengthen your vessels and arteries and help revive your sluggish responses. Your blood pressure will soon level off at a healthy balance.

Enjoy a healthier life span with a healthy blood pressure, made possible through everyday power foods!

See CHOLESTEROL, CIRCULATION.

BODY ODOR
Power foods that eliminate this embarrassment

Perspiration is a healthy function. Also known as sweating, it is a normal means of regulating your body temperature. When you become too warm or overheated (this occurs throughout the year in all temperature ranges), your skin signals your brain-located thermostat to direct more blood to the surface of your body (to your skin capillaries). There is an increase in the release of fluid (perspiration) from your sweat glands. As your perspiration evaporates, you feel cooler.

Perspiration is passive transudation of almost pure water from your body surface at a constant rate. The water immediately evaporates. But at the same time, either the moist or dried perspiration (or both if the process continues throughout the day and/or night) will become acrid and give off an unpleasant odor. This is known as body odor. It can be unpleasant, embarrassing, even if the sweating process is nature's way of keeping you cool and cleansed since waste products are being removed. You may bathe regularly, but there still may be a disagreeable odor. This is caused by action of bacteria on the stale sweat.

To help mask and even remove body odor, a program for external and internal cleanliness with the help of power foods will make you more pleasant to others and to yourself, too.

POWER FOODS TO HELP ELIMINATE BODY ODOR

Cleansing-Deodorizing Herbal Tea. Brew a tea of the herb, vervain. (Available at most health stores and herbal pharmacies.) Use one teaspoon to one cup freshly boiled water. Add a bit of honey and fresh lemon juice for flavor. Let steep five minutes. Sip slowly. Drink three freshly prepared cups per day.

Benefit: Vervain contains an herbal ingredient that tends to induce perspiration and cleanse your system of offending wastes. This helps you look and feel fresh, clean and naturally deodorized!

Masks Skin Odors. Brew a tea of the herb, fennel. (Available at health stores or herbal pharmacies.) Use one teaspoon to one cup freshly boiled water. Flavor with a bit of honey and fresh lemon juice. Let steep five minutes. Sip slowly. Drink two freshly prepared cups per day.

Benefit: Nutrients in fennel appear to mask odors released from perspiration. You will feel much more refreshed even if you do perspire because fennel tea acts as a natural deodorant.

Green Leaves. Green leafy vegetables are prime sources of magnesium, a mineral that combines with calcium and phosphorus to activate better carbohydrate metabolism and for maintenance of body temperature, muscle contraction, and nerve impulse transmission. These are the metabolic processes involved in perspiration. It is magnesium that causes an internal washing as it deodorizes the elements involved in these processes. So you perspire but there is a refreshing reduction in odor.

Power Food Program: Daily, eat a large raw green salad with lemon juice and vegetable oil for a dressing. You will be giving an abundant magnesium supply to your metabolic system so it will be washed and deodorized as it cools you off. Magnesium may well be a natural deodorant!

Body Refreshing Tonic. Blenderize lettuce leaves, celery stalks, turnip greens, cabbage and any other seasonal green leafy vegetables. Drink one glass in the morning. Drink another glass of this *Body Refreshing Tonic* in mid-afternoon. The high concentrate of magnesium will be empowered by the catalytic action of the enzymes to wash out wasteful substances from your body but, at the same time, mask the odor. You will then feel refreshed and more youthfully healthy.

POWER FOODS THAT ARE NATURAL DEODORANTS

You can make these power foods at home with everyday ingredients. Apply them as deodorants and they will take away offensive odors.

Odor-Away Powder. Combine equal parts of powdered cornstarch (or arrowroot powder) with boric acid. Dust under your arms with this powder. This *Odor-Away Powder* fulfills its name by eliminating the odor, and helps you keep dry at the same time.

Lettuce Odor-Ease. In a wooden bowl, crush romaine lettuce leaves. The juicier and more succulent they are, the more beneficial they will be. Mash until some liquid appears. (You may want to blenderize the romaine leaves into a juice.) Apply the liquid to your underarms or just splash over your perspiring body. The darker the leaves, the darker the juice. This indicates a prime source of chlorophyll, a plant juice that helps do away with odor.

Cucumber Control. Slice a very juicy, very large cucumber in half. Rub the juicy half over your perspiring body parts. Squeeze the cucumber half as you do so that the juice will wash and then dry on your skin. In a little while, the offensive odor is gone—and it stays gone for many, many hours. The high magnesium content of the cucumber acts to block and then dilute the acrid substances responsible for the odor. It helps rub off skin debris and wastes. A youthful skin texture is the healthy result.

Mild Foods = Better Health + Odor Freedom. Strong body odors are often traced to an intake of very sharp, spicy and volatile foods. These include harsh spices, strong onions and garlic as well as an excess of meat foods. Metabolic wastes from such foods are strongly odorous. Change to milder foods. They are less strenuous on your metabolic system. They improve your health because they do not demand strong digestive action. Milder foods will also give you more freedom from body odor.

Perspire because it's healthy to do so. Use power foods to eliminate embarrassing odor because it's healthy to do that, too!

See FOOT PROBLEMS, SKIN.

BONE AILMENTS
Power foods that strengthen your skeleton

A well-nourished skeletal structure will resist the shock of fracture-causing falls, the fragility of osteoporosis, the softness of osteomalacia.

Nutritionally strengthened bones will also give you better body shape and support, and more protection for your internal organs. Power foods contain nutrients that can give girder-like strength to your body skeleton so that it will resist great pressures, yet be flexible enough to absorb a certain amount of shock without shattering—as, for instance, when you trip and fall. A strong skeleton will help resist the impact so that while you may experience bruises, you minimize or eliminate the risk of a fracture. With the use of power foods, your skeleton can become strengthened so that your body is protected against such physical shock.

THE EVERYDAY BEVERAGE THAT FEEDS YOUR BONES

An everyday beverage, available at almost all food stores, is a powerhouse of minerals that will feed your bones and give them strength and resistance against weakness.

That beverage is *milk*. A powerhouse of calcium and phosphorus, this power food works to feed your bones and replace minerals that are lost through the daily process of metabolism. During the routine of digestion, bone minerals are being torn down and rebuilt through the blood flow between the skeleton and the rest of your body. This same digestive process sends a large supply of calcium to the matrix, or spongy matter in the cavity of the bones. But this same mineral, along with phosphorus, is needed for the contraction of muscles, the beating of the heart and blood clotting. If the calcium and phosphorus available for these functions drop below a certain level, your blood now takes them from your bones. If you are deficient in these minerals, your bones become drained and fragile and problems of weakness occur. Any pressure or slight injury may cause breakage.

To help give your metabolism an abundant supply of these bone-building minerals, you need milk daily. This power food contains ample amounts of these minerals together with skeleton-strengthening Vitamins A and D to help build a strong bone structure to support your entire body.

From "Weak Bones" to "Young Body" in Seven Days. Librarian Hazel N. tripped while standing on a small footstool attempting to remove books from a high shelf. She experienced a sharp pain on her side, and needed help to get up and move to a chair. The pain persisted. Her examining physician said she had very "weak bones," a condition similar to that of osteoporosis (also known as "brittle bones"). In this condition, Hazel N.'s skeletal structure became porous because of a loss of calcium and phosphorus. She did complain of back pain, a chronic aching in her spine. She had rounded shoulders. Her doctor told her to follow a simple program which was that every single day, she was to drink three glasses of mineral-rich milk. This everyday beverage provided a rich supply of the needed bone-building minerals so that her skeleton could be strengthened to resist impact. Within seven days, Hazel N.'s condition went from "weak bones" to "young body." She continues to drink at least two glasses of this "bone tonic" as she calls it and is no longer troubled with back or spine pain. Her shoulders straightened out. She walked with the posture of a much younger woman. Later, when she tripped and hurt her hip, she had some bruises, but no bone injury. With the help of mineral-rich milk, her skeleton had become young and strong and break-resistant!

THE POWER FOOD THAT BUILDS YOUNG BONES

Daily, take four tablespoons of this easily available power food to help build a strong and young skeletal structure. This power food is *cod liver oil.* It is a dynamic treasurehouse of Vitamins A and D which are needed to help protect the body against the problems of osteoporosis and osteomalacia, forerunners of brittle bones and hazardous fragility.

Vitamin Benefits of Cod Liver Oil: The essential Vitamins A and D are used by your metabolism to give rigidity to your bones, to correct softening and improve the density or volume. This protects against bone aging that is caused by osteoporosis and osteomalacia. In these conditions, there is a marked vitamin deficiency characterized by softening of the bones, a diminishing of bone density that may lead to crumbling. The vitamins are needed to boost absorption of dietary calcium so that tiny spaces in the bone center are able to become strong enough to support the surrounding bone tissue. Vitamins A and D create this strengthening reaction with the help of calcium.

Cod liver oil, available at health stores and most pharmacies, is a powerhouse of these important bone-building vitamins.

Young Bone-Building Tonic. In a glass of any desired vegetable juice, stir two tablespoons of cod liver oil. Flavor with a bit of lemon juice, if desired. Drink one glass at noontime, and a second freshly prepared glass at dinnertime. You will be sending a stream of powerful bone-building Vitamins A and D into your metabolism so that within seven days, your skeleton will become youthfully strengthened. It's the tasty way to build strong, young bones along with a young body, too.

Boost Bone Health with Sunshine. To protect against bone fragility, try to treat your body to as much sunshine as possible. (Do not overdo this as it may cause skin burning.) Get out into the fresh air and sunshine whenever possible. When natural sunlight strikes your skin, the ultraviolet portion stimulates a lipid substance, 7-dehydrocholesterol, just below the surface, to form cholecalciferol (Vitamin D_3). This substance nourishes your bones, gives them strength, helps protect against problems of osteoporosis and osteomalacia. Just 60 minutes (not all at one time) daily will create this metabolic reaction that works almost immediately to boost bone health. It is the natural and totally free power food from nature!

With the help of such everyday power foods as milk, cod liver oil and warm sunshine, your body skeleton can become strong and healthy so that you will feel youthfully vigorous.

See ARTHRITIS, NECK PAINS, SPINAL COLUMN, STIFFNESS.

BREATHING DIFFICULTIES
Power foods that open new air channels

Throughout the year, many folks are troubled with breathing difficulties. In cold weather, bronchitis as well as colds afflict more and more victims. There are choking spasms, stuffed noses, wheezy breathing. In warm weather, allergies ranging from asthma to hay fever cause running noses, sore throats, reddened and watery eyes, a feeling of total misery. The "breath of life" is so precious that if it is denied for longer than a minute, the body is thrown into a feeling of panic! In the middle of the night, if there is a choking spasm, the entire respiratory tract reacts and the feeling is that asphyxiation will bring on the end of life! The muscles that control breathing feel paralyzed and shock worsens the problem as the fear is that fatal choking is taking place. To help improve your powers of respiration, various foods are available, along with simple but effective daily living programs.

HOW TO DRINK A GLASS OF "FRESH AIR"

Troubled with breathing difficulties ever since he could remember, Thomas J. would awaken at night, choking and coughing. He would run to the window to breathe in fresh air. His throat was always parched and irritated from constant coughing and sputtering. He felt resigned to this problem. A physiotherapist told Thomas J. that he needed to rebuild his weakened bronchial-respiratory system. He needed to boost his intake of Vitamin A. He told Thomas J. to take this simple tonic at least three times daily:

In a glass of carrot juice, stir one tablespoon of any fish liver oil (cod, halibut or shark), together with one tablespoon of desiccated liver (available at health stores and most pharmacies). Stir vigorously. Drink one glass in the morning, another freshly prepared glass at noontime and a final one before bedtime.

Thomas J. was so desperate for air, he was willing to try any program that promised breath restoration. He followed this easy program for five days. He was amazed! He could breathe better. Gone were the late-night choking spasms. He no longer had to sputter and choke. He felt, as he put it, that he had been "drinking a glass of fresh air."

Benefits of "Fresh Air" Tonic: The carrot juice, fish liver oil and desiccated liver are triple sources of powerful Vitamin A. When taken as a tonic, the vitamin works speedily. It helps preserve the healthy physiological functions and anatomical structure of the mucous membranes. It also goes to work to regenerate and restore the destroyed membranes. Therefore, these membranes are now able to release a substance called *lysozyme* which acts to destroy harmful bacteria. This "Fresh Air" Tonic provides this important Vitamin A that reconstitutes your respiratory organs so that you can breathe better in a short time.

SAY GOODBYE TO BRONCHIAL DISTRESS WITH CITRUS POWER FOODS

Inflammation of the bronchial tubes is caused by bacterial or viral infections. Bronchitis usually occurs in winter or when the climate is wet and cold. But it is also experienced during warmer months because of the problem of increasing air pollution, cigarette smoking and overcrowded living conditions. Breathing difficulties are often traced to malnourished or weakened bronchial tubes. To say goodbye to this type of distress, build resistance with the help of citrus power foods.

Oranges, Grapefruits, Tangerines Are Lung-Building Power Foods. These citrus fruits are powerhouses of Vitamin C, a nutrient that can so revitalize your breathing apparatus in a short time that you will be able to say goodbye to bronchial distress and enjoy healthy fresh air at all times.

These power foods are able to promote the healing of damaged bronchial cells and build up a barrier against infectious germ invasion. They also work to build up antibodies (disease fighters) in your bloodstream to neutralize toxins and give your entire bronchial system a natural immunity to infections and ailments. These power foods send Vitamin C directly to your main air tube (the trachea) to strengthen and invigorate this source of inhalation so that you can breathe more easily and more healthfully. The power foods also send Vitamin C to your bronchioles, or smaller tubes, to give them more flexibility, to help dispose of wastes that may cause clogging and enable you to breathe with enjoyment.

Breathe Easier with Citrus Elixirs. Daily, enjoy Citrus Elixirs in the form of pure orange, grapefruit or tangerine juice, either singly or in any desired combination. These juices are available in all food markets. You may want to squeeze or blenderize your own. Plan to drink at least three glasses daily for powerful Vitamin C, needed to regenerate your bronchial system so you can breathe easier.

Try a Citrus Fruit Salad Daily. Begin each meal with an assortment of citrus fruit wedges (remove seeds) on a bed of lettuce leaves. Use a dressing made of lemon juice and oil. Chew thoroughly. You then release the Vitamin C from the fibers so it can be assimilated speedily to help repair the cellular components of your breathing components.

Drink and eat citrus fruit daily for more breathing power!

THE POWER FOOD THAT UNBLOCKS CONGESTION—IN SECONDS

Europeans have long been able to open up "blocked" channels with the use of an everyday power food. It costs pennies but provides priceless help—in a matter of a few seconds. That power food is ordinary *horseradish*. This volatile flavoring contains pungent substances that create a volatile reaction when inhaled. All you need do is fill one tablespoon with horseradish, then slowly inhale. You will feel the congestion loosening up and disappearing within a few seconds. Just a few inhalations will help you breathe easier and better and end your choking spasm. Keep a bottle of horseradish by your bedside to use for inhaling if you should awaken in the middle of the night with frightening choking spasms. It is a power food that has been used for many centuries as a natural breathing aid.

TO BREATHE BETTER FOLLOW THESE HELPFUL PROGRAMS

1. Give up smoking. Nicotine congests the delicate membranes of your respiratory passages. Avoid areas that are smoke filled.

2. Avoid extremes of heat or cold. Sudden abrupt changes play havoc with your respiratory reflexes and may bring on a choking attack. Going from the hot outdoors into an air-conditioned cold indoors (or vice versa) may trigger off this breathing problem. Give your body a little while to adjust to the change by holding a clean handkerchief to your nostrils and breathing in warmed air before making any change.

3. Keep hands and feet comfortably warm. Do not let them chill since blood is drawn away from your respiratory tract in an effort to keep your extremities warm, and this causes breathing distress. If you feel chilled in bed at night, wear woolen socks and gloves, too.

4. Instead of caffeine-containing coffee and tea (which may cause acceleration of your heartbeat, intensification of your blood pressure and bronchial congestion), switch to fruit and vegetable drinks, coffee substitutes such as Postum and herb teas. Avoid cola beverages. Not only do they contain caffeine, but they are taken ice cold and this can bring on a bronchial spasmodic reaction.

5. Use natural herbs and spices as seasonings instead of salt. The reason is that the sodium portion of salt becomes stored in the skin, the mucous membranes and other bronchial tissues and reduces the ability of your breathing organs to provide you with a steady supply of fresh air. Avoid salt in cooking and in the shaker.

6. Shower or bath water should be comfortably warm or cool. Extremely hot or cold water causes a change in your rate of respiration, making you breathe more rapidly. This forced respiration removes much of the carbon dioxide from your circulation without

replacing it with oxygen, and this brings on disorders of the respiratory tract.

With the help of power foods that are eaten, drunk or inhaled and with changes to improve your daily lifestyle, you should be able to unblock clogged breathing channels and enjoy much-needed nutritious air!

See ALLERGIES, ASTHMA, COLDS, COUGHS, EMPHYSEMA, SINUSITIS.

BURNS
Power foods that cool pain and speed healing

All burns are serious. They may be fractional (when you touch a hot stove and leap away) or of longer duration (when you broil yourself under the hot sun). With some simple protective measures, you can build your body's resistance and insulate yourself against the pain and the scarring risks of any burn. You may also use everyday power foods to help cool the pain and speed the healing of most burns.

WATER: SOOTHING POWER FOOD

Cold water is a time-tested power food that is able to bring immediate relief to the pain of a burn. As soon as you feel the pain of a burn, immerse the afflicted part in water as cold as possible. If this is impossible to do, pour cold water over the area that has been burned. You will feel relief almost immediately. Follow through by cutting away loose clothing. Cover with several layers of cold moist dressing. (Do NOT remove clothing adhered to skin.) Seek medical aid if the burn is extensive.

Quick Help for Chemical Burn. (1) Flood affected area with water for at least 20 minutes until all chemical is removed. (2) Remove all clothing because chemical may be retained in the garment and cause further irritation. (3) Do not break blisters. (4) Do not use ointments. (5) Seek medical aid promptly.

THE RAW JUICE WAY TO SWIFT HEALING OF BURNS

Any burn, however mild, causes a form of shock. In this situation, blood pressure drops to a serious low. There is a loss of body fluids which then rush to nourish the injured body part. The rest of the body is consequently deprived of liquid, and this may cause shock.

To correct, fortify yourself with several glasses of fruit or vegetable juices. In particular, citrus fruit juices are essential because they are concentrated sources of Vitamin C which is needed to help build collagen, the cement-like substance that heals, knits, binds cellular tissues together. Furthermore, a plentiful supply of liquids in your body at the time that there is a loss through reshifting of fluids to cool the burned area will also minimize the reactions of body shock. As soon as the burn has been cooled with water, drink fruit or vegetable juices to protect against body dehydration.

Ordinary Drinking Water Is a Power Food for Burn Healing

When you receive a burn from any source, the body reacts by pushing potassium out of your injured cells. Your body also releases sodium from your bloodstream to be excreted. In order to replace the loss of sodium, your bloodstream turns "cannibal" by taking this mineral out of its own reserves to be sent to your cells. This causes a serious blood pressure drop, kidney weakness and dizziness. You need to replace the lost sodium in a hurry. You do this by following this amazingly simple but effective power food program:

Drink two or three glasses of ordinary tap water as soon after the burn as possible. Nearly all water contains *natural sodium* (as opposed to chemicalized sodium chloride from a salt shaker), which helps replenish that which is lost. Just two or three glasses will send sufficient amounts of sodium to your cells. Now potassium will return, being magnetized or drawn to the sodium. Your bloodstream is spared its self-depletion of needed natural sodium and your entire body is able to function more healthfully. Once the essential sodium-potassium-water balance is maintained, burns are cooled and healed much more rapidly.

VITAMIN E: POWERFUL HEALER OF BURNS

Any burn will destroy tissue. If serious enough, it may even leave a scar. To help protect against this risk, follow this simple program that utilizes Vitamin E, a nutrient that soothes the pain, but sends forth a form of balm that heals up the jagged edges of the cells and promotes swifter and smoother healing so there is less (if any) scarring.

Break open the contents of several capsules of 500 international units of Vitamin E, apply to a clean gauze cloth, and use as a bandage upon the burned area. The alpha-tocopherol ointment is natural and soothing and works almost immediately. Change the dressing daily until you see healing and pain is gone. It may help protect you against the threat of permanent scarring through the knitting of the burned skin cells. Vitamin E capsules are available at all health stores and pharmacies.

Cooling Severe Burns in a Hurry. Make a paste of water and ordinary baking soda. Spread over the burned area. Let remain at least 60 minutes. When dry, splash off in a tepid bath.

Power Food Burn Ointment. Mix one cup buttermilk with two peeled, mashed tomatoes. Spread this ointment over the burned area. The minerals in these two power foods are especially soothing and cooling. They help take the sting out of a severe burn in a matter of minutes. Let remain for 60 minutes, then rinse off under tepid water.

Yogurt-Tomato Burn Healer. It's good enough to eat and apply to your burn, too. Combine one cup plain yogurt with the strained juice of two tomatoes. Apply to the burned area. Let remain at least 60 minutes. Rinse off with tepid water or under the shower. The fermented milk tends to energize the minerals of the tomato juice to provide speedy nourishment to the injured skin tissues and help create cooling repair very speedily.

Act quickly to cool pain and speed healing of burns with these power foods—taken internally and used externally. Your skin will be glad you did.

See SKIN.

BURSITIS
Power foods that unlock congestion and soothe pain

A bursa is a sac (pouch-like space) lying between two structures, such as between bone and skin, bone and tendons, etc. Whatever irritates a bursa—a mineral deposit, a blow on the side of the hip, the improper grip on an object (tennis racket, broom, screwdriver)—may produce a pain. This is known as bursitis, or housemaid's knee, tennis elbow or painful shoulder. Because the most common area is the bursa about the shoulder, bursitis usually strikes this particular region. It can, however, affect other joints such as the knees. Floor scrubbing or any task that calls for much movement on the knees may irritate the bursa in the lower limbs and bring on an attack. It can last for a few moments or can be more severe and cause intensive pain for hours or even days. In severe situations, it may cause disabling.

FOUR POWER FOODS THAT SOOTHE PAINFUL BURSITIS

Janice Y. was troubled with recurring bouts of bursitis. After doing much housework, she would develop such painful shoulder spasms that she had to lie down and rest for several hours. Other times, Janice Y. would experience a wrenching pain if she reached up to a high shelf. Just lowering her upstretched arms would cause pain. She brought her bursitis distress to a local health clinic. The healer explained that sluggish metabolism had led to congestion of elements in the bursa and that their breaking up would be required in order to enjoy relief and freedom from the pain.

Janice Y. was told to boost her intake of four special power foods: wheat germ, bran, brewer's yeast, liver (whole or desiccated). She was told to use these four foods daily. She followed the clinician's suggestions for nine days. Gradually, she noticed that her shoulder pain was diminishing. Now she could move her arm in full range with hardly any spasms or shock tremors of pain. At the end of the nine days, she was so healed that she could do a full day's work without any pain in her shoulder—or anywhere else, for that matter. Now she continues eating these four power foods daily and enjoys freedom from bursitis.

Benefits of the Four Power Foods: These foods (wheat germ, bran, brewer's yeast, liver) are highly concentrated sources of Vitamin B_{12}, a little-known but highly effective power food that helps unlock bursitis congestion and soothe pain. These four power foods, taken together or singly, are prime sources of both Vitamin B_{12} and folic acid which work together to create a synthesis of nucleoproteins. This metabolic reaction tends to break up the cluster of elements in the bursa sac and redistribute them, restoring mobility to the joint. These two vitamins stimulate improved, youthful metabolism of nervous tissue, bringing about pain relief of irritated nerves in the area. Within a few days, these power foods have released sufficient amounts of Vitamin B_{12} and folic acid to restore a balance of elements in the body and thereby cleanse the affected bursa sac of its irritants. This promotes a powerful healing reaction that makes life more worth living with more youthful energy and vitality.

How to Use These Power Foods. Daily, use wheat germ, bran, brewer's yeast as part of whole grain cereals, sprinkled over raw fruit or vegetable salads, in soups, stews, casseroles, baked goods, even as a tasty breading for chicken, turkey, meats, vegetables. Use desiccated liver in the same way. Or add two tablespoons of this highly concentrated B_{12}-folic acid bursa cleanser to a glass of tomato or carrot juice. Stir vigorously. (Blenderize for better assimilation.) Drink two glasses daily. Prepare broiled liver and onions for this same high nutrient value and eat at least twice a week. You will be giving your metabolism the needed nutrients that help break up stubborn accumulations of substances that grate inside your bursa sac. Your metabolism will use these nutrients to dislodge the substances, break them up, then release them from your body. Your cleansed bursa sac will then have greater and more youthful mobility. Plan to use these four power foods daily. When pain has diminished, use them frequently to protect against recurrence of bursitis.

PAMPER YOUR SHOULDER FOR REDUCED PAIN, MORE COMFORT

Be good to your painful shoulder joint (or any area where bursitis-like pain is felt) and you should be able to relieve and eliminate the distress.

Basic Problem: Every movement, however slight, causes friction which in turn causes a spasm of pain. You cannot remain immobile because this causes sluggish circulation-metabolism and worsens the condition. You need to use caution when making body motions.

Basic Health Tips: Train yourself *not* to work or hold your arm too long in difficult positions. Shift from your right to your left arm as frequently as possible. If you have to open a door, lift up a fork, hold a book, push an object, brush your hair, clean your teeth, even scratch yourself, use the well arm and let the ailing arm rest a little bit. Apply contrasting hot and cold compresses to the ailing area every night. For just 15 minutes, apply a comfortably hot compress (let it remain until it cools), then a comfortably cold compress (let it remain until it becomes warm). This alternating hot and cold application will help loosen up congestion and promote better flexibility of your arm. Painful deposits may also break up and be redistributed and eventually excreted through this home remedy, used along with the four basic power foods outlined above.

ICE: HEALING POWER FOOD FOR BURSITIS PAIN RELIEF

When painful bursitis strikes, reach for some ice cubes. As a power food (ice is made from water which is a food!), ice produces the feeling of cold which tends to numb the inflammatory pain. Be prepared. Put ice cubes in a plastic refrigerator bag or ice bag, wrap in a towel and apply to the painful region for 15 minutes. Now remove for 15 minutes. Then apply again. Continue this ice healer for one hour or longer. It is this contrast of cold and room temperature that helps to dislodge accumulated pain-causing crystals and free them for eventual removal. Have ice cubes ready and waiting in your freezer at all times for speedy use and quick healing of distressful pain.

Be sure to swing your arm in every direction when you are free from distress. Do this gently but regularly. If you restrict movements, then you may develop disabling adhesions which will cause the joint to become stiff and even paralyzed because of disuse. Keep your arm (and body) active. Use power foods and power remedies. Your bursitis can then be relieved and you'll be able to unlock congestion and enjoy pain-free arms and legs. You'll look and feel flexible and young again!

See ARTHRITIS, BACKACHES, MUSCULAR ACHES, NECK PAINS, SPINAL COLUMN, STIFFNESS.

CHEST PAINS
Power foods that untie knots and calm flutters

Chest pains are frequently caused by excessive exertion, emotional upset, eating a heavy meal, or sudden exposure to extreme cold from temperature or foods and drink. They may come on suddenly and last a little while, or may be mild at first, increase in intensity and last for a long time.

Such chest pains are usually felt in the center of the chest behind the sternum (the flat bone in the center). The pains may radiate to a shoulder and travel down to the elbow or wrist. Ordinarily, such pains are not sharp but are squeezing, gripping, constricting sensations.

In some situations, you may feel palpitations, dizziness, shortness of breath. You may break out in a cold sweat. Such chest pains may be symptomatic of angina pectoris, which is nature's way of urging you to seek medical aid. Frequently, chest pains are the consequences of errors in daily living—that is, subjecting your body to such mischief-causing non-foods as sugar, salt and an excess of animal fats. Other errors include the intake of alcohol and tobacco, improper rest, unrelieved tension, physical and/or mental overexertion. These abuses are responsible for knots and flutters that react in the form of chest pains.

Basic Pain-Soothing Programs. Eliminate all forms of sugar and salt in cooking as well as from the shaker. Read packaged products. If they contain these non-foods, better pass them up. Reduce intake of animal fats. Cut off all visible fats before cooking meats. Cut off any remaining fat before eating. Quit the drinking and smoking habits. Enjoy a full night's sleep. Reduce your daily obligations so that you do not feel physically or mentally exhausted. With these self-pampering programs, you will be soothing your circulatory-respiratory systems so that you will have less strain and fewer (if any) annoying knots and flutters.

THE SWEET POWER FOOD THAT EASES CHEST PAINS

A deliciously sweet food that is golden in color offers a gold mine of natural power to help ease and erase recurring chest pains. That power food is the *banana.* It is a prime source of many important nutrients, especially *potassium*. It is this mineral that has the power to correct body disorders, establish healthy equilibrium and restore soothing comfort to your chest as well as other systems and organs.

Power Food Benefit: When you eat the tasty banana, you give your metabolism an abundant supply of potassium. Almost immediately, this mineral works with sodium in the extracellular fluid to regulate blood pH (acid levels that may cause chest pains if imbalanced), body water balance, acidification of urine so that irritants can be eliminated through waste channels. The banana potassium becomes involved in soothing nerve conduction and muscular contractions. It then helps regulate the required equilibrium between the intra- and extracellular fluid. This corrects body disorders, and when the fluid levels are properly balanced, the chest pains subside and disappear. A power food bonus of the banana is that its highly concentrated potassium supply will help wash away muscular weakness and fatigue and create a feeling of vitality and energy, often within a short time. The naturally sweet banana offers a powerhouse of potassium-building health and longer life. All this with good taste, too.

Pain-Soothing Banana Shake. Mash one ripe banana with a

fork; combine with one cup fruit juice. (Orange or grapefruit is recommended.) Blenderize for one minute or until smooth and creamy. Drink one glass in the morning, a second glass at noontime, and a third glass after your evening meal.

Benefits: The Vitamin C in the fruit juice will catalyze the potassium of the banana and propel it speedily through your system. Now this mineral is able to create speedy healing of disorders and ease and erase chest pains. The Vitamin C-energized potassium will nourish the muscles of your chest so that contractions are soothed. Nerve conductions become more relaxed. You will feel very content. Within 30 minutes after taking this tasty *Pain-Soothing Banana Shake*, your chest pains should subside. You'll soon feel good (and glad) all over!

THE HERB TEA THAT CALMS YOUR CHEST FLUTTERS

A cup of freshly brewed *peppermint* tea, flavored with lemon juice and a bit of honey, is an amazing power food that can calm your chest flutters within minutes. The peppermint herb is a highly concentrated source of many vitamins and minerals, notably the valuable potassium and magnesium. These are needed to restore body equilibrium so that chest pains can be soothed and knots untied almost immediately.

How to Prepare Peppermint Tea. Use one teaspoon of this herb (available at most health stores, herbal pharmacies, supermarkets) to one cup boiling water. Let steep for three minutes. Add a desired amount of lemon juice and honey. Sip slowly. Plan to enjoy this calming tea at least three times a day.

Benefits: The peppermint plant offers you a powerful supply of magnesium. This power mineral is used for mobilization of calcium from the bones to create a feeling of calmness and relaxation. Muscular contractions that are painful may be crying out for magnesium which is made available with peppermint tea. This power mineral functions as a co-factor, helping enzymes in metabolizing many biological reactions so that there is internal stabilization of fluids and less incidence of waste accumulation which may cause discomforting chest and body pains. Plan to drink peppermint tea regularly. It's the tasty way to enjoy freedom from chest pains.

By making a few adjustments in your daily living program, by using these power foods, you should be able to enjoy a healthier and longer life without recurring chest pains.

See ASTHMA, BREATHING DIFFICULTIES, CIRCULATION, MUSCULAR ACHES, STIFFNESS.

CHOLESTEROL
Power foods that wash away excess body fat

Perhaps the single most important risk factor for arteriosclerosis, heart problems, and blood pressure irregularities is a high blood level of lipids (fats), particularly cholesterol. This fat is a compound that is needed by the body—but in modest amounts. It is an important part of the nerve tissue. It opposes elements which would ordinarily destroy red blood corpuscles. It reduces the wateriness of cells, giving them a semi-solid character. Cholesterol is indeed important to your health—in the right amount.

A problem is that when it increases too much, accumulates in places where it does not belong, it can cling to the walls and interiors of the arteries, become weighty, cause clogging and reduce the free transport of air and nutrients and thereby create a risk to your health and life. Because cholesterol is introduced into the body through animal fats, it is suggested that a reduction of these foods would help protect you against cholesterol overload.

Cholesterol Sources at a Glance. You should know that cholesterol is found ONLY in foods in animal origin. These include all meats, dairy products, eggs, and products made with these foods. Cholesterol does NOT appear in foods of plant origin such as fruits, vegetables, grains, seeds, nuts and products made with these foods. To self-regulate your cholesterol intake, just be aware of these basics about this fat.

You Need Some Cholesterol. Going on a totally cholesterol-free food program is unwise. Although your body manufactures some of this fat, you still need it from animal foods—but in limited and controlled amounts. Cholesterol is required for the manufacturing of glandular hormones, the formation of cell-tissue membranes, the creation of brand new cells and tissues. Cholesterol is a structural element in cell walls and the sheaths around certain nerve fibers called myelin sheaths. Cholesterol is also converted chiefly to bile acids that aid in your digestive processes. So this fat is needed—but in amounts that your body can safely handle. It is when you take in more cholesterol than your metabolism can break down that you have the *overload principle* that could be injurious to your health and take years off your life.

In helping your body cope with cholesterol, and in helping your metabolism digest any excess and restore fat-balance in your organism, various power foods are especially beneficial.

EGGPLANT: POWER FOOD THAT WASHES AWAY BODY FAT

The glimmering, satin-polished eggplant contains a nature-balanced supply of vitamins, minerals and fiber that is able to help prevent cholesterol from accumulating within your body. These substances go to work almost immediately after you eat the baked or cooked eggplant and act as a barrier to block accumulation of excess fat or cholesterol.

Power Food Benefit: Digested eggplant releases its elements which tend to bind up fatty cholesterol in the intestine, "capturing" it and then transporting it out of your system before it can become assimilated within your bloodstream. It is this anti-absorption power of eggplant elements that gives it this power food benefit. In effect, eggplant elements become the brake on the cholesterol train and call a halt to its runaway escape into your body.

Suggestion: Enjoy eggplant regularly, whether in the form of a vegetable steak, as a casserole, with cheese or with meat, or as a relish. It's an effective fat-fighting power food.

HOW ONIONS TAKE THE STING OUT OF CHOLESTEROL

The common onion is a prime source of potassium along with Vitamin A; the two work in harmony to help dislodge accumulations along the walls of the arteries. When onions are eaten, these nutrients are able to attack the clumps of cholesterol and with the use of the volatile oils present in this power food, help break down even the most stubborn of plaques and then prepare them for elimination. The natural carbohydrates of the onions will energize your metabolism so that there is an acceleration of the processes needed to remove accumulating cholesterol.

Suggestion: Feature sliced, chopped, diced onions regularly as part of a salad. Use onions either boiled, stewed, baked or sauteed as a flavoring of most of your meals. Try an omelet with onions and chopped green peppers.

The active principle in onions is not destroyed by heat and is not water soluble so you may use this wonder food either raw or cooked. It is a tangy way to take the sting out of cholesterol.

LECITHIN: HIGH-POWER CHOLESTEROL MELTING FOOD

Lecithin is a food derived from soybeans. It is available in granule form at most health stores and pharmacies. Its power food benefit is that it helps to emulsify or homogenize cholesterol in the body. By loosening cholesterol deposits, it keeps your arteries and heart cleansed and protected against any excess.

Power Food Benefit: Lecithin contains lipotropic agents which are needed to metabolize fat. As a phosphatide, it is an essential component of all living cells and tissues. It acts as a "keeper of the gate" in that it protects the cells and tissues from an invasion of excessive cholesterol. Lecithin is particularly powerful in lowering the surface tension of aqueous solutions. The reason is that one side of the molecule prefers fat, while the other is attracted by water. This unique action makes lecithin an effective emulsifying power food, capable of dissolving excessive cholesterol deposits.

Suggestion: Use lecithin granules as part of a salad dressing; add them to whole grain cereals. Add several tablespoons to tomato juice and drink one or two glasses daily. Supplements are available.

Lecithin Creates Healing Miracle. Ralph L., a 45-year-old baker, was troubled by chest pain and could not work. The doctor who examined him noted he had yellowish-brown plaques under his eyes. He also had a high (almost abnormal) cholesterol level.

The doctor gave Ralph L. a low-cholesterol and low-fat diet and also gave him prescribed amounts of lecithin. Within two months, Ralph L.'s chest pains were gone. His cholesterol level was lowered appreciably. His fatty plaques (xanthalasma) vanished from his face. He now felt completely healed and could enjoy a longer life span as he returned to work, thanks to lecithin!

Control cholesterol supplies with the use of power foods and you will keep your arteries and heart youthfully clean.

See ARTERIOSCLEROSIS, CIRCULATION.

CIRCULATION
Power foods that energize circulation

A throbbing circulation is symbolic of youthful health. When you are able to energize your circulation and keep it moving throughout the day, you will be able to enjoy the most that life has to offer. A vitality-filled circulation may well be the key to better health and longer life.

With the use of simple but amazing effective power foods, you should be able to wake up your sluggish circulation and invigorate its components so that it soars through your body, giving you the feeling that life is beautiful.

Your blood vascular circulatory system is responsible for uninterrupted delivery of oxygenated blood and its energy-producing nutrients to all of your billions of cells and tissues. This same system promotes cellular exchange of waste products of metabolism, then transporting those wastes to points of elimination. No body system has a more serious responsibility than your circulatory system for without a supply of oxygenated blood, your cells and tissues would soon wither and die.

If your circulatory system is sluggish, these cells and tissues may survive—but on the borderline between health and bare survival. Therefore, the benefit of power foods is that they give your circulatory system an energy boost, take up the slack, and establish a healthy rhythm so that it can give you youthful energy throughout the day.

THE VEGETABLE OIL THAT BOOSTS YOUR CIRCULATION IN MINUTES

Cold-pressed from whole grains, wheat germ oil has the amazing power to supercharge your sluggish circulation, help cleanse your bloodstream of wastes, and promote a youthful "push" to give you immediate vigor and energy. Wheat germ oil, when taken by the spoonful or added to vegetable salads or mixed in a juice, is a powerful circulation-booster.

Oxygen Regulation = Circulation Increases. Wheat germ oil contains alpha-tocopherol, also known as Vitamin E, which is able to create oxygen regulation in your system and bring about a healthy circulation increase. This vegetable oil uses Vitamin E to control blood viscosity or thickness which slows the circulation and creates congestion in your system. Wheat germ oil will take Vitamin E, transport it through your blood circulation, help wash out sludge from your bloodstream. This increases the amount of oxygen made available to your body cells and tissues. All organs become energized and your entire body responds with youthful health and a longer lifespan. At the same time, wheat germ oil will use Vitamin E to prevent the oxidation or destruction of essential fatty acids in the blood and this creates an important oxygen regulation that promotes more youthful vitality. The action of wheat germ oil is virtually immediate so that within moments after taking it, your body responds with better energy.

With Circulation Boosted, She Feels Much Younger. Lillian F. was in her early 50's but she looked and acted as if she were in her 70's. Her skin had a pale, sickroom pallor. Her breathing was labored. Climbing up just a few steps would leave her gasping for air. When Lillian F. went shopping, she felt exhausted after waiting on a line for only a few minutes. She was always wanting to sit down, no matter where she went. She was aging too fast. An orthomolecular physician (specialist in nutritional healing) heard of her fading energy and suggested she take at least 16 tablespoons of wheat germ oil daily. Lillian F. tried a simple program as outlined. Within two days, she began to look and feel more youthful. Her skin started to glow. She breathed with youthful energy and could walk and stand without feeling constant fatigue. Lillian F. felt the years roll back; after one week on this simple program, she looked younger than her early 50's. She continues taking wheat germ oil daily, calling it her "youth medicine."

Circulation-Boosting Program. Use wheat germ oil as part of your salad dressing. Add four tablespoons to tomato or carrot juice, stir or blenderize, then drink slowly. Add to soups, stews, casseroles, baked goods. Plan to use at least 16 tablespoons daily for effective circulation boosting.

Benefits: The Vitamin E in the wheat germ conveys oxygen from your lungs to your billions of body cells. Then it transports carbon dioxide from your tissues back to your respiratory system where you exhale it regularly. The same Vitamin E works instantly to transport nutrients from your digestive-intestinal system through your liver to your fatigued tissues to energize and revive them. The Vitamen E will also transport waste substances from your tissues to your organs of elimination, thereby creating internal cleansing of toxic wastes, often the cause of fatigue. It is this revitalization of your internal organs that makes wheat germ oil a miracle worker in boosting circulation and giving you youthful vitality and better health.

WHOLE GRAIN FOODS: CIRCULATION ENERGIZERS

Whole grain foods such as wheat germ, bran, rye, oats, in the form of breads, cereals, baked loaves or stews are prime sources of a little known but powerful circulation booster. A member of the B-complex vitamin family, this energizer-booster is *folic acid*. By eating a small portion of whole grain foods daily, you send a powerfully concentrated amount of folic acid through your digestive system to create almost immediate circulation energizing.

Power Food Benefit of Folic Acid. If you are troubled with constant fatigue, weakness, a feeling of heaviness across your shoulders, then take advantage of this power food. Whole grain foods with folic acid can revitalize your body and mind, often within 60 minutes, so that you will feel vigorous and healthy. Folic acid has a unique power to create vasodilation of the smaller blood vessels.

Once these channels are opened by folic acid, this power food provides a supercharging of hydro-dynamic pressure so that a wider route is made available for transmission of blood. Through this circulatory route, the oxygen- and nutrient-carrying blood will energize your billions of body cells and tissues. In effect, it is like creating dynamic vitality within your circulatory system. By expanding your blood vessels, folic acid creates a miracle of rejuvenation since the key to better health and longer life is in a network of sufficiently wide vessels. Folic acid is the power food that can create this burst of vitalic energy within a short time.

Morning Circulation Booster: Put one cup of any desired whole grain cereal (read label to see it contains no additives) in a bowl and add orange or grapefruit juice. Sprinkle with whole grain wheat germ and bran. Add desired sliced fruits. Sun-dried raisins are concentrated sources of energy-boosting so should be used regularly. Just one bowl of this *Morning Circulation Booster* will revitalize your body/mind network and you'll feel supercharged with vigor for nearly half the day.

Benefits: The folic acid of the whole grain cereal is triggered by the energizing factors of the Vitamin C in the fruit juice and then doubly invigorated by the fructose of the raisins. In moments, this energy is dispersed throughout your body, alerting your sluggish circulation so that you have that "glad to be alive" feeling. It will show in your youthful activities and your glowing face. It's the tasty way to start the day off with vim and vigor—and keep going the rest of the day, too.

Wake up your sleepy circulation with these power foods and discover how it feels to be young again!

See Cholesterol, Weakness.

COLDS
Power foods that promote healing and build your natural immunity

Yearly, in cold and even mild weather, people catch colds. Sneezing, coughing, sputtering, feelings of weakness, sore throats, runny noses are only a few of the annoying symptoms that may last for a day or a week or even longer. Colds are annoying. They may force you into unwanted bed confinement. They keep you isolated from others who do not want to catch your cold. Yet, no matter how many medications you take, you still continue catching colds. The reason is simple:

A cold will invade your body when your resistance is too weak to keep out the infectious germs. There is no chemotherapeutic cure for colds. The only way to resist colds and to promote healing when you have been infected is to give your body the working materials with which it can destroy the infectious invaders.

Power Foods or Chemical Foods? Various power foods contain substances that can destroy the *cause* of the cold and thereby create effective healing without risky side effects. Chemical foods are able to suppress the symptoms and mask the discomfort, but cannot destroy the infectious organism or give you that much-desired natural immunity; they also may have undesirable side effects considering that you are already suffering with the ailment. For better healing and for possible natural immunity, power foods seem to be the practical answer to the problem of cold-catching.

VITAMIN A: FIRST LINE OF DEFENSE FOR HEALING AND IMMUNITY

Because infectious germs penetrate the mucous membranes of the naso-pharnyx throat linings, it is important to strengthen this first line of defense against colds. Vitamin A has the power to preserve the health of the mucous membranes. It aids in the regeneration and restoration of these membranes when they become injured or destroyed. Vitamin A rebuilds the cilia (microscopic hair-like covering of the membranes) and energizes it so that it can sweep foreign matter, such as cold-causing germs, toward the pharynx where it can be discharged. Vitamin A preserves the strength and health of the mucous membranes and replenishes these cells when cold germs have attacked them. To build your powers of healing and natural immunity, boost your intake of Vitamin A.

Cold-Fighting Power Tonic. To a glass of carrot juice, add one tablespoon of cod liver oil, one tablespoon of desiccated liver (from health store or pharmacy), one teaspoon of honey. Blenderize for one minute. Now drink slowly. Plan to drink at least four glasses of this *Cold-Fighting Power Tonic* each day, from the start of any symptoms until you are healed.

Benefits: The carotene from the carrot juice is transformed into usable Vitamin A that is then combined with the nutrients in the oil, strengthened by the protein and vitamins in the desiccated liver. In this form, it has more stability and a "time release" reaction because of the slow absorptive character of the honey. One glass gives you a gradual deposition of Vitamin A and you have prolonged healing and buildup of immunity. In many situations, you can be healed within one day with the use of this *Cold-Fighting Power Tonic.*

Other Sources of Power Vitamin A: Fresh liver, most fish liver oils, kidneys, egg yolk, cheddar cheese, butter, milk, broccoli, sun-dried apricots, cantaloupe, leafy green vegetables.

HOW TO DRINK YOUR WAY TO FREEDOM FROM COLDS

Whether you have a cold or whether you want to build natural immunity, take advantage of the nutrients in citrus juices. When prepared freshly, they are powerhouses of Vitamin C, one of the most effective cold fighters currently available.

Citrus Juices Work Speedily. The juice of any citrus fruit (orange, grapefruit, tangerine or lemon) is more rapidly digested than is the fruit itself. While you should eat fresh citrus fruits daily because they are high concentrates of cold-fighting Vitamin C, you should use their juice for swift healing and immunity. Pressed juice is more easily absorbed by your digestive-metabolic system for more rapid assimilation which is needed when you have a cold. At the slightest sign of what you think may be a cold, start drinking at least four glasses or one quart daily of these citrus fruits, either singly or in any desired combination.

Needless to say, lemon juice is unpalatable to drink by itself. But use a few tablespoons in any citrus fruit juice you prepare. Lemon juice is a powerhouse of cold-fighting Vitamin C.

Benefits: Vitamin C in the citrus juices (and fruit pulp) has the power to heal wounds, prevent cellular destruction, and help build a barrier against germ invasion. These power food juices contribute to the building up of disease-fighters or antibodies in the bloodstream. *They also neutralize toxins in your bloodstream, and that is the secret of their ability to give you natural immunity to infectious colds.*

Eat and drink Vitamin C-rich citrus fruits daily and your body will have the working materials required for healing and immunity to colds.

Garlic: Powerful Cold Fighter. A European remedy for many centuries, garlic is one of the most effective cold fighters available. To help heal a cold, use chopped or diced garlic with a raw salad that includes parsley to mask its strong odor. Garlic contains sulfides and disulfides. These compounds attach themselves to virus matter and thereby inactivate them, so their cold-causing powers cease. If you start chewing and eating garlic early enough, your cold may be healed within a matter of hours! You should also eat garlic often throughout the year to create natural immunity to infectious germs. It is a powerful natural antibiotic!

Basic Cold Healing Health Tips

If you feel an approaching cold, begin by using the power foods recommended for swift healing and eventual immunity. You should also follow these common-sense health tips to speed recovery:

1. Your food program should consist of lots of fresh fruits, vegetables, their juices, whole grains, low-fat protein, seeds, nuts.
2. Stay home and rest. You needn't be bedridden (unless your cold is serious) but you should limit activities. Keep yourself warm. Avoid temperature extremes.
3. Keep a moist indoor atmosphere. Your respiratory system will utilize the power food nutrients more effectively in a moist climate. You may want to use a small vaporizer near your bed.

With the use of power foods and common sense, your cold

should respond to swift healing. Your body should be rewarded with immunity to the common cold if you follow basic programs.

See Allergies, Asthma, Breathing Difficulties, Coughs, Fever.

COLITIS
Power foods that correct intestinal disorders

An irritable colon can create total body irritation because it leads to a drain on the vital nutrients needed to maintain good health. In colitis, there are variations from diarrhea to constipation, ranging from mild to severe. In diarrhea, the loss of nutrients can cause serious deficiencies throughout the body. In constipation, the accumulation of toxic materials can create a form of internal toxemia which can cause erosion of important organs as well as destruction of billions of cells and tissues.

Except for the common cold, colitis is believed to be the most common disorder of man.

Basically, colitis is a nervous ailment that strikes stress-filled people. Often, the disorder is triggered off by some stimulus such as emotional upset, physical strain, hasty eating or drinking, unrelieved stress. The colon (large bowel or intestine) reacts to such situations with variations from diarrhea to constipation.

If neglected, the condition may worsen to become ulcerative colitis in which there is swelling of the mucosa, internal skin sores, loss of elasticity. Colitis should be corrected as swiftly as possible to help control loss of important health- and life-building nutrients.

THE POWER GRAIN THAT CORRECTS COLITIS IN A FEW DAYS

Bran, an everyday grain, has the power to help correct most intestinal disorders, including colitis, in a matter of days. This power food has the ability to create digestive homeostasis or healthy balance within a short while.

What Is Bran? Bran is the indigestible, structural part of the outer layers of the wheat kernel. It is composed of complex carbohydrates including cellulose, hemi-cellulose, pectin and lignin, a woody substance.

How Does It Heal Colon? As a power food, bran provides bulk that absorbs moisture and helps your digestive system keep clean. This power food prompts your intestinal system to self-regulate its own activities.

What Are Its Powers? Bran hastens the removal of waste matter in constipation and thereby protects the intestinal canal from putrefactive bacteria. Bran also nourishes the colonic cells and muscle tissues so that they become self-regenerated to guard against diarrhea. This power food acts directly on the intestinal microflora, either inhibiting or removing the production of colitis-causing substances.

How Does It Revitalize Colon? This power food increases the moisture content and bulk of the stool, which in turn dilutes the concentration of potential toxic substances. Bran thus blocks their contact with the intestinal wall, creating a shield that protects the colon from harmful substances. This helps the colon strengthen itself and become youthfully revitalized.

FREEDOM FROM COLITIS IN FIVE DAYS WITH SIMPLE POWER FOOD

Embarrassed by colitis, Henry O'C. had tried a variety of different chemical remedies. They worsened his problems that varied from loose to clogged bowels. He kept getting weaker as a result of lost or improperly metabolized nutrients due to this organ distress. Henry O'C. was fearful of leaving his home when he was troubled with colitis because he thought he would have an "accident" while in the street or on a bus. This made him so nervous that his problem increased. Because he was unable to go to his local pharmacist to pick up his medication, the druggist called to ask about his health. Henry O'C. said that nothing seemed to help control his colitis. The pharmacist recommended the use of simple bran. Available in every supermarket or health store, as well as at pharmacies, it was reportedly a power food that would strengthen the ailing colon so it could self-regenerate and heal itself. The program was simple: take ten tablespoons of bran daily, either with a whole grain cereal, or divided up in soups, stews, casseroles, blenderized with fruit and vegetable juices, most baked goods. This would help rebuild the colon. Henry O'C. tried this program and in five days experienced such relief from a revitalized colon that he began to enjoy youthful vitality and energy. His bran-healed colon gave him better health and hope for a younger life span.

THE JUICY POWER FOOD THAT REBUILDS A SLUGGISH COLON

Recurring bouts with diarrhea and constipation can weaken the muscular walls of the colon, rendering it less effective in its function as an elimination channel. To rebuild the colon, a juicy apple is an appetizing power food. This tasty fruit is a prime source of pectin, a cell-tissue healing substance that is needed by the components of the walls of the colon. When you digest a well-chewed apple, you send a supply of hemicellulose to your fluttering colon to nourish its muscular frazzles and rebuild its worn-out segments. Eating apples daily will help create youthful functioning of your digestive-regulatory-eliminative systems. These healed chain links will boost the strength of your colon and it will be able to perform its daily function of youthful regularity.

Colon Detergent Benefit. Well-chewed apples are used by your digestive system to create a catalytic action upon your colon. The pectin and hemicellulose of the metabolized apples will create a mild fibrous action upon the internal organs, such as the colon, using a detergent effect to help wash away accumulated toxic wastes that impede normal function. The apple will also provide much needed bulk to help correct the problem of constipation. As a power food, the apple should be enjoyed daily. It is the natural way to correct intestinal disorders through colonic revitalization.

Be good to your colon (and your body) by cutting down on emotional stress and avoiding excessive physical strain. Take time to eat and drink. If you feel tensed up, then just relax. Don't work or eat until you feel soothed. It's good for your colon and your body, too

With proper care and the enjoyment of simple power foods, you should be able to correct intestinal disorders and be rewarded with better health and a longer life.

See CONSTIPATION, DIARRHEA, DIGESTIVE DISTURBANCES, DIVERTICULOSIS.

CONSTIPATION
Power foods that give you natural regularity

Afflicting folks of all ages and all walks of life, constipation is an ailment that automatically calls for the use of chemical remedies. Habitual use of such patent concoctions will weaken the intestines and they will be unable to function on their own. It thus becomes a serious or vicious cycle. The habitual use of laxatives can cause constipation. Dependence upon these synthetic methods can reduce the muscular contraction force of the intestines until prolonged or chronic constipation is the result. There is accompanying mental anguish because something has gone wrong with the body.

When Is Constipation Serious? If there are at least three days between bowel movements and the passage of very dry stools, then the condition is serious. An occasional skipped day is no cause for alarm, however. *Problem:* Excessive straining at stools among the elderly can often precipitate a heart attack or stroke. Therefore, constipation for folks in the middle years should be treated promptly. A rule of thumb: never strain at bowel movements, regardless of your age!

THE ROUGHAGE WAY TO SMOOTH ELIMINATION

Roughage is found in a group of power foods that will help end the problem of constipation almost immediately. Roughage is coarse bulky food that is very high in fiber. By its bulk, roughage stimulates peristalsis, successive waves of involuntary contraction passing along the walls of the intestines to create smooth elimination.

Roughage Power Foods. Whole grain breads and cereals provide roughage. These should be made from unbleached whole wheat, bran, rye, barley, buckwheat, oats, hominy grits, corn meal, soybean flour, millet. These power foods will help provide the necessary bulk to induce a natural elimination. Plan to eat several slices of whole grain bread in the morning. You should also eat a whole grain cereal with some fruit. The fruit will energize the roughage of the grains to create needed bulk, often within an hour. Pancakes, waffles, muffins, rolls, should also be made of this whole grain flour. Many of these products are available in supermarkets and most health stores. Read labels. They should be stated "whole grain," which is your key to unlocking internal congestion.

Raw Vegetable Power Foods. Carrots, fibrous lettuce, cabbage, cauliflower, celery, tomatoes, green peppers, red peppers and radishes are powerful sources of roughage to help create a natural bulk. Plan to eat an assortment of these fibrous vegetables daily so that you will be able to energize your sluggish bowels and induce natural regularity.

PRUNES: NATURAL LAXATIVES

The humble-looking prune is a power food without comparison as an all-natural laxative. The prune provides soft bulk and has the vitamin and mineral content that make for the intestinal muscle tone essential for good body elimination. The prune contains an active principle that performs specifically as a regulator of the large intestine. The prune will provide a gentle, safe stimulation that makes chemical laxatives unnecessary and prevents the dire results which often follow their use.

Eating a plateful of pitted prunes in the morning, then drinking a glass of energizing orange or grapefruit juice, will help start the bulk-forming process that will induce a natural movement, often within 30 minutes. As a power food, prunes may well be the number one natural laxative!

FIGS: THE NATURALLY GOOD INTESTINAL POWER FOOD

Revitalize your sluggish intestines with the use of figs. The secret here is that during the ripening process of figs, the natural sugar content rapidly increases. These simple sugars (monosaccharides), in the form of dextrose and fructose, are the simplest and smallest carbohydrate molecules requiring no digestion since they are absorbed directly into the bloodstream from the intestine. These natural fruit sugars provide powerful energy that regenerate your sluggish intestines so they can perform almost immediately!

Eat a bowl of figs in the morning (combine with pitted prunes for double-action power) and drink a glass of citrus fruit juice. Within moments, your powerfully energized intestines will "wake up" and perform smoothly. You will be able to conquer constipation with this power food without any delays.

Power Food Juice. Prune and fig juice, singly or in combination, can work speedily to alert your intestines in the morning so that they can function youthfully. Drink one or two glasses upon arising, *on an empty stomach* so there is no interference from other ingested foods, and you'll have a "power food juice" that offers both bulk and liquid to create natural movements—within moments!

BRAN: NATURAL BULK-FORMING POWER FOOD

Much of constipation can be traced to dryness. This is where bran comes in. You have probably chewed raw wheat germ or natural bran and noted the slippery quality that develops when chewing. This is the moisturizing property that is the key to the power of bran in easing constipation. When you eat bran, it remains unchanged by your digestive fluids and passes down your entire digestive tract unchanged. Thus it lubricates your dry intestinal wall.

Specifically, bran is hygroscopic in that it retains moisture in the intestinal waste. Through lubrication and moisture retention, it helps build up natural bulk.

Bran has a supply of minerals and cellulose which stimulate the musculo-nervous mechanism of the intestine, increasing the propulsive force that moves the intestinal waste out of the system. By eating sufficient bran daily, you provide your bowels with the roughage that stimulates muscular activity to create regularity. Bran also offers minerals that will both stimulate and support nervous control of those muscles to keep them working efficiently for regularity.

Use bran daily by sprinkling it over your favorite whole grain cereal. Add bran to any prepared food such as soup, casseroles, meat or fish dishes. Sprinkle it on top of fruit or vegetable salads.

When baking, just leave out a little of the flour and replace it with bran. You'll discover that your intestines soon become invigorated and before long you will soon enjoy healthful and natural regularity.

With the use of these everyday (and tasty) power foods, your body will bounce back to youthful vigor and health and life will become refreshingly good.

See Colitis, Diarrhea, Digestive Disturbances, Diverticulosis.

COUGHS
Power foods that soothe throat irritations

An irritated sore throat provokes a cough which is nature's way of helping your body rid itself of infectious material. Occasional coughing is not serious, especially if the itching, scratching feeling is relieved when you sip a cool beverage. But if a cough persists, it may suggest a serious problem which should receive prompt attention.

In general, coughing will be caused by irritation of the pharynx (area in back of the throat) which may be traced to excessive use of your voice, the swallowing of irritating foods (hot spices, red pepper, alcohol), dusty working and/or living conditions, smoking, or the inhalation of industrial and environmental pollution. Many coughs are caused by colds so the method of relief would be to heal the cold. In more serious situations, swallowing is difficult and there is a feeling of heavy mucus which is difficult to clear away.

To help soothe your irritated sore throat, correct the causes listed above. Foods and beverages should be mildly flavored; avoid volatile spices. Quit smoking and drinking. Avoid others who do because the vapors and odors emanating from them may irritate your naso-pharynx region, prompting a coughing spell. Clean up your environment so you will have less exposure to throat irritants. Keep away from areas that may fill your lungs with dust or noxious fumes. Seek out well-ventilated places, wherever you go.

To help soothe a cough-irritated throat, there is one totally free power food that works wonders within moments.

WATER—THE COUGH-SOOTHING POWER FOOD

As a food, water is totally free, available for use in almost any circumstance and powerful enough so that it can relieve your cough almost immediately.

Here are five ways in which you can use water to bring speedy and welcome relief for your cough:

1. *Enjoy Water.* Drink it straight from the tap or use bottled spring water. It's soothing and speedily effective and enjoyable if you sip slowly. You'll also boost your needed water intake by means of hot or iced herb tea (sip slowly). Fruit drinks are powerhouses of Vitamin C and water which work together to heal and lubricate your parched throat.
2. *Disperse Water.* A humidifier will increase the amount of moisture dispersed in the air. You can also give your throat much-needed extra moisture simply by covering a radiator with a wet bath towel. In just a short time there is more moisture in your room and your throat feels better.
3. *Drink Water.* Several eight-ounce glasses of water every day will give your body much of the water it needs to thin out phlegm and moisten dry, inflamed tissues of your mouth, nose and throat.
4. *Eat Water.* Most fruits and vegetables are 80% water. Eat them daily. Fish is 75% water, meat and eggs 50% water. By eating these foods, you'll be providing your body with soothing moisture.
5. *Inhale Water.* In the form of steam, it is throat-soothing, cough-easing. An electric vaporizer converts water to steam and is most helpful at your bedside. A teakettle on an electric plate will also give you much needed and throat-welcome water.

Importance of This Power Food. Habitual coughing causes much loss of water through increased perspiration and evaporation due to heavier breathing. That is one reason why you should use this power food, water, to replace that which is lost. Another important benefit is that this power food will help your cough bring up the mucus that is formed in your respiratory passages. Water helps keep the mucus thin and liquid and helps the cough do the job nature intended. Finally, water and humidity can make you more comfortable until the cough subsides and goes away.

POWER FOODS TO SOOTHE SORE THROAT AND HEAL STUBBORN COUGHS

Here is a compendium of time-tested power foods that help soothe and relax the reflex muscles involved in cough production and help heal your irritation.

- Roast a ripe lemon in your oven until it cracks open. Now take just one teaspoon of this lemon juice with a quarter teaspoon of honey. Take the same amount every 30 minutes. You should feel relief almost immediately.
- Gargle several times a day with this cough-healing power food combo: combine one pint of boiled water and four tablespoons of apple cider vinegar. When it is comfortably cool, use it to gargle with. Repeat a few times. The cough should be soothed and gone within one day.
- Antiseptic oils in a garlic clove are helpful in nullifying the harmful irritation of infectious bacteria lodged in your throat tissues. Just chew and swallow one garlic bulb daily. To mask the strong odor, munch on some parsley leaves at the same time.
- Moisturize and lubricate your throat with this power food formula: mix cooked barley with some lemon juice and water. Eat with a spoon. The grain oil with the tart lemon juice will help overcome toxic bacteria and soothe your frazzled throat, often within 30 minutes.
- Chronic coughing will often cause a hoarse throat. This creates further irritation and more coughing. To end this vicious cycle, try this healer: mix a small amount of grated horseradish with some honey and eat with a spoon. Just two teaspoons every three hours will help detoxify your throat, soothe the irritation, and end your coughing problem.
- To nip coughs in the bud, try sipping dill tea (available from health stores and many herbal pharmacies). Just add one teaspoon of dill to one cup of boiled water. Flavor with a bit of lemon juice and honey. Just three cups during one day should help make the cough go away—and stay away!

A healthy throat will build a strong and youthful respiratory system. Treat it well. Soothe it with power foods when troubled with coughs. You'll soon be able to breathe better, speak better and live much better (and longer), too!

See ASTHMA, BREATHING DIFFICULTIES, COLDS, EMPHYSEMA.

CRAMPS
Power foods that relax-soothe stomach unrest

The digestive system reacts sharply to physical and/or mental abuse. When you take in food or beverages that are scalding hot or ice cold, the esophagus (food gullet or passageway for food from mouth to stomach) reacts by contracting or expanding rapidly. This causes an outpouring of hydrochloric acid (digestive juice) that tries to cope with the shock of the unwelcome intruders. The stomach further rebels at this flooding of excess juices and this causes what is known as acid stomach, sour stomach, or an annoying stomachache. Cramps may be mild, making you wince, or they may be so severe that you cry out with pain. You want speedy help. Should you use bicarbonate of soda?

Cramp-Causing Penalty of Bicarbonate of Soda. The answer is a resounding NO! This antacid, taken by itself or as part of a patent remedy, will neutralize stomach acid and ease the cramps. But it also becomes absorbed through the walls of your stomach and this worsens your acid problem. Furthermore, the use of bicarbonate of soda causes your digestive organs to release more acid and this compounds the problem. Therefore, the relief you get is momentary and then backfires as the bicarbonate of soda causes more cramps.

Yogurt: Power Food for Fast Cramps Relief. Reach for a cup of plain yogurt when troubled with stomach cramps. This is a *fermented* power food. It is a powerful source of an all-natural cramp-conquering substance known as *Lactobacillus acidophilus*.

This powerful substance produces large amounts of lactic acid as it feeds on lactose from dairy products.

Benefit: Lactic acid is a powerful destroyer of ache-producing harmful bacteria. By crowding out and eventually expelling unwanted bacteria, the lactic acid is able to restore soothing comfort and also boost production of needed B-complex vitamins that soothe frazzled digestive organs.

Ache Relieved in 60 Minutes. Barbara I. was constantly troubled by recurring stomachaches. She tried bicarbonate of soda but noticed that while the knife-like pains subsided quickly enough, they returned a little while later with more severity. She was so troubled with the acid burning sensation that she could barely eat or drink anything. Complaining to the public health nurse in her factory building where she worked as a secretary, Barbara I. was told to eat just one cup of plain yogurt whenever she felt the threat of an ache. She was advised to eat and swallow slowly. Desperate, Barbara I. had a cup of yogurt. Amazed, she told the nurse that her cramps vanished within 60 minutes after finishing the yogurt. More important, the ache did not return. Now, whenever she feels the threat of an ache, she enjoys this power food, yogurt. To build immunity to aches, she has this power food once daily. It's the refreshing way to enjoy freedom from stomachaches.

Power Food Beverage That Calms Down an Outraged Stomach

Warm and soothing, a cup of freshly brewed lavender tea, flavored with a bit of lemon juice and honey, will help calm down an upset stomach. This herb (available at health stores and herbal pharmacies) contains emollient oils that are released into the water as it steeps. When sipped, these oils tend to coat the frazzled digestive organs, acting as a soothing anointment so that the irritations start to subside. Sip comfortably warm tea whenever you feel the onset of a stomachache. It should work almost immediately.

WASH AWAY STOMACHACHE WITH A GREEN POWER JUICE

Select any seasonal lettuce, borage, celery, or a combination of whatever is available. Wash the leaves. Put them in a blender, add some water, then whizz at medium speed until of a smooth consistency.

Now, drink this *Green Power Juice* as soon as you feel any spasm or warning of an ache. Drink slowly. Drink one or two glasses. Within 15 minutes, your ache will subside and you will feel peaceful contentedness.

Benefit of Green Power Juice: The green vegetables, high in vitamin-mineral content, are empowered by their enzymes to send soothing comfort to your digestive organs. This unique juice has a mucilaginous effect and coats the organs with a comforting film which protects against corrosive elements. In just a little while, you will feel the ache going away and the burning sensation will disappear. Takes minutes to prepare . . . takes minutes to heal!

SEVEN WAYS TO PROTECT YOUR STOMACH AGAINST ACHES AND CRAMPS

Be good to your stomach, avoid abusing your digestive organs, and you should be able to enjoy an ache-free lifestyle. Here are seven ways to help you protect yourself against annoying cramps:

1. *Limit Sighing*. Yes, habitual and repeated sighing leads to *aerophagia* (excessive air swallowing) and this causes your digestive system to become pressure filled and react by protesting with aches. Keep air swallowing to a minimum. Train yourself not to breathe in through your mouth.
2. *Eat in Comfort.* Do not gulp down your food. Neither should you eat if you are emotionally or physically upset. Your digestive organs tighten up and food cannot be properly handled. This may cause serious aches. Wait until you are totally relaxed before you eat, even if it is just a small item.
3. *Drink Slowly.* Do not wash down any liquids in a hurry. Neither should you wash down foods during or at the end of a meal. This causes air-buildup, and gas bubbles trying to escape will cause an ache. Drink slowly from a cup or a glass. Keep your upper lip submerged by tilting the cup. Do not use a straw as this, too, causes excessive intake of air.

4. *Basic Tips.* Avoid carbonated beverages as they have air bubbles which cause digestive upset. Avoid foods that have air whipped into them such as whipped butter, porous breads or cakes, any so-called milk shakes. *Never* drink hot beverages since you will instinctly gulp in air to cool off your throat. This, too, leads to a stomachache.
5. *No Smoking, Please.* Tobacco boosts the flow of oral (mouth) saliva: an excess of saliva will increase your swallowing and this, in turn, automatically increases air swallowing. Give up smoking and your stomach (as well as the rest of your body) will be healthier.
6. *No Air Swallowing, Please.* You may feel the urge to swallow air in order to bring up pain-causing gas bubbles—but this is a vicious cycle. More air is swallowed than is brought up. Therefore, you intensify or add to the problem. It's like adding more fat to a fire. Don't swallow air!
7. *Be Regular.* Correct problems of constipation through the means of bulk-forming raw grains, fruits, vegetables, nuts, seeds. Having regular movements will help clear away toxic wastes that may be causing stomachaches. A clean colon will help keep the rest of your body healthy and ache-free, too.

At the first warning sign of a stomachache, reach for a power food instead of a chemical. You'll feel glad you did!

See DIGESTIVE DISTURBANCES.

DIABETES
Power foods that boost natural insulin release

Diabetes is caused when cells in the pancreas known as the islets of Langerhans fail to produce the hormone *insulin.* (The pancreas is a large, long organ or gland located behind the lower part of the stomach.)

A deficiency of insulin means that the body is unable to metabolize carbohydrates (sugars and starches). Sugar (or glucose) now accumulates in the blood until it spills over into the urine. This continued loss of essential carbohydrates will cause diabetic symptoms. These include excessive thirst, hunger, urination. Weight is constantly lost, despite increased food intake. The body grows weak. Skin disorders are common. Vision is blurred. The legs feel tingling cramps. Diabetes worsens if it is neglected as the blood glucose level starts to seesaw.

Synthetic Insulin May Cause Reactions. Doctor-prescribed insulin is supposed to provide that which the pancreas is not manufacturing in sufficient quantities. But this may have adverse effects. Insulin shock may be caused by too much insulin getting rid of too much sugar at one time. Facial swelling and vision distortion are just two of the most common side effects caused by synthetic insulin. Yet the body does require an adequate amount of insulin to help metabolize sugars and starches. A sluggish pancreas needs to be alerted and activated so that it can perform healthfully, releasing an adequate amount to cope with these carbohydrates.

BREWER'S YEAST: POWER FOOD FOR YOUR LAZY PANCREAS

To help your body handle sugar, to nourish and activate your lazy pancreas so it will release normal amounts of insulin, one particular element is needed—*chromium.* This trace element (mineral) acts as a supercharger in that it enters the delicate islets of Langerhans distributed throughout the pancreas and alerts and activates them so that they can release more insulin.

Chromium is found in a highly concentrated form in a power food known as *brewer's yeast.* This power food consists of the dried, pulverized cells of the yeast plant. It is a very powerful composite of highly concentrated nutrients, especially that of chromium. (It contains *no* sugar, *no* fat, almost *no* starch, making it most beneficial to the carbohydrate-watching diabetic.) The chromium in the brewer's yeast tends to regulate the delicate mechanism of the islets of Langerhans in the pancreas, resulting in a controlled and time-release secretion of natural insulin.

Basic Benefit: Insulin cannot function without chromium which may well be the most essential mineral needed by the pancreas. When supplied with a high concentration of chromium through brewer's yeast, the pancreas is better able to function in its task of releasing sufficient insulin. The glucose levels of the blood tend to rise together with the chromium, since both need one another to maintain a healthy balance. Chromium is bound in an organic form in the glucose tolerance factor and thereby helps regulate insulin release and utilization.

Pancreas Activating Power Tonic. To boost the insulin-making powers of a sluggish pancreas, nourish it with chromium. Try this *Power Tonic:* In a glass of tomato juice, add two tablespoons of brewer's yeast (available at health stores and pharmacies). Stir vigorously or blenderize a minute. Drink one glass in the morning, another glass at noontime and a third glass in the evening. You may want to drink more throughout the day. Use other vegetable juices such as cabbage, celery, lettuce, etc., for a variety in taste.

Within moments after it is swallowed, the chromium from the brewer's yeast is released into the bloodstream where it is able to enter the islets of Langerhans, latch onto insulin components and speed the hormone to all parts of the body where it will digest sugars and starches. Because brewer's yeast is such a highly concentrated source of this mineral, it is considered a power food.

Other Power Foods for Chromium. These include liver, beef, whole wheat bread, beets, mushrooms. While these foods contain appreciable amounts of chromium, you would need to eat large quantities in order to obtain an adequate amount of this power mineral. Therefore, it is more effective to use brewer's yeast, which speeds a dynamic "power" of chromium to your pancreas to alert it to release needed insulin . . . in a short time.

THE HERB THAT CREATES NATURAL INSULIN

The yarrow herb is believed to contain the active components of insulin, biologically speaking, and it should be taken as a tea as often as possible. To prepare: add one teaspoon of yarrow flowers (from health store or herbal pharmacy) to one cup of freshly boiled water. Let steep five minutes. Add desired lemon juice and honey. Plan to drink several freshly brewed cups of yarrow herb tea daily. It will help boost insulin manufacture.

BLUEBERRY LEAVES FOR DIABETIC CONTROL

If blood sugar levels are too high, healers recommend the use of blueberry leaves. (Not the berry itself, but the leaves, which are available from herbal pharmacies.) As a power food, blueberry leaves brewed as a tea release an active principle known as *myrtillin* which helps produce excess sugar in the blood.

To Prepare: Steep blueberry leaves in a pot of freshly boiled water for 20 to 30 minutes. Flavor with lemon juice and honey. Drink several cups throughout the day. Plan to brew a fresh infusion each time since the *myrtillin* principle evaporates or loses potency if not taken fresh.

By controlling your glucose tolerance levels with this tea, you stimulate your pancreas to release sufficient amounts of insulin.

THE POWER FOOD MINERAL THAT ACTIVATES THE PANCREAS

Manganese is a trace element that often determines whether or not the pancreas will release sufficient insulin. This mineral is so powerful that it influences glucose metabolism and regulates glucose tolerance. It stimulates the pancreas so that it releases sufficient insulin to utilize excess carbohydrates.

Power Benefit: Manganese is required for the synthesis of acetylcholine, which is a neurotransmitter that sets off pancreas action so that insulin pours forth to cope with carbohydrate metabolism.

Sources of Power Mineral: Green leafy vegetables, whole grains, brewer's yeast, herbs such as cloves, ginger, cardamom. Also available as a supplement.

Wake up your sleepy pancreas with these power foods and help your body properly utilize carbohydrates to protect against insulin deficiency.

See Digestive Disturbances, Low Blood Sugar, "Sweet Tooth."

DIARRHEA
Power foods that control and correct irregularity

Also known as loose bowels, diarrhea is a condition in which there are frequent or excessive bowel movements. Diarrhea is a symptom of a disorder that has taken place either in the bowels or elsewhere in the body. Causes range from overeating, food poisoning, bacterial infection, abuse of laxative drugs, emotional stress, fatigue, even a reaction to climate change. In particular, excessively hot weather may bring on diarrhea since the body is trying to cope with the harsh climate and does so by severe relaxation of many organs, including the bowels. This brings on a loose discharge. The body tries to cleanse itself of toxic bacteria as speedily as possible. If diarrhea is mild, lasting only a few hours, it calls for a period of rest and improved nutrition to replace essentials that have been lost. If it continues for several days, it is serious and should receive prompt attention.

POWER FOODS THAT HELP CONTROL DIARRHEA

Basic Benefit: The power foods suggested in the following paragraphs have a unique benefit. They are able to "bind up" the foods that you eat so that they do not slide through your intestines so rapidly. By providing a natural "brake," they halt diarrhea. This gives your body an opportunity to absorb nutrients of eaten foods.

Simple, Quick, Effective. Because of the solidifying quality of these power foods, and their rapid digestibility, they are simple to take, work swiftly and create this binding effect upon the loose bowels within a very short time. These power foods are miracle healers for problems of diarrhea.

Chopped Apples + Cinnamon = Speedy Diarrhea Control. Chop or dice two washed and cored apples. Sprinkle with a bit of cinnamon. Eat slowly, and be sure to chew thoroughly before swallowing.

Healing Benefit: The fibrous-containing pectin of the chopped apple unites with the cinnamon to create a carminative effect upon the slack bowels. Both of these power foods act as astringents, helping to tighten up loose muscles; they also act as a carminative in that they help remove from the intestines harmful bacteria that may be responsible for the diarrhea. The fibrous pectin acts as a solidifying agent, further boosted by the tree-bark-created cinnamon to tighten and bind up looseness and bring about control and correction of this irregularity.

Bananas: Sweet Way to End Diarrhea. Natives of the tropics in Central and South American appear to be immune to diarrhea, often called "Montezuma's revenge" or "touristas." Their secret of bowel health may be their use of the local banana. Now you can use this secret to help control and correct your own bowel irregularity. Whenever you have this condition, however mild, eat a few bananas. Take no other food or beverage. Within two hours, your bowels should be strong enough so that you need not keep running to the bathroom.

Healing Benefit: The secret of the anti-diarrheal action of the banana power food is in its unusual tree-ripened pectin which tends to swell when digested and bring about voluminous, soft stools. Because this tree-ripened power food is a high source of natural fruit sugars, it is speedily digested and metabolized, therefore the reason for its swift effectiveness, often within 30 minutes. The banana tends to absorb unhealthy bacteria while inducing the growth of bowel-strengthening organisms. This restores bowel balance and helps correct irregularity. Rich in potassium, along with other minerals, the banana will replace minerals that have been lost in diarrhea, thereby strengthening the intestinal organs and the entire body, too. For any diarrhea problem, reach for this golden fruit of the tropics. It's the native's secret for freedom from diarrhea.

Plain Yogurt Is a Natural Power Food Healer. Joseph D. usually eats on the run, finds it difficult to relax, travels around from one part of the country to the other, subjecting his body to many climate changes. Frequently, he develops diarrhea. A public health nurse once told him that when he feels the slightest symptoms, he should take plain yogurt with some wheat germ, if desired. Nothing else. This helps control and correct this irregularity. Joseph D. follows this advice and rarely has diarrhea. If it does strike, it is the plain yogurt (two or three cups within an hour) that promotes speedy and powerful healing.

Benefit: Yogurt, as a fermented milk product, is a powerhouse of *Lactobacillus acidophilus,* a beneficial bacteria that becomes established in the colon and strengthens its muscular contractions so that the looseness is firmed up and diarrhea subsides. This works very swiftly so benefits are enjoyed within a short time. If you add wheat germ or bran, the roughage content will further firm up the loose bowels so that they become corrected even faster.

With the use of these everyday power foods, diarrhea can be eased and eliminated. The entire body can then respond with better health and more youthful vitality.

See Bladder, Colitis, Constipation, Cramps, Digestive Disturbances, Diverticulosis.

DIGESTIVE DISTURBANCES
Power foods that cool "burning" and energize metabolism

Youthful health and longer life depend upon a healthy digestive system. Foods ingested must be properly metabolized and their nutrients thoroughly assimilated in order for your body glands, organs, systems to become invigorated and strong enough to help you enjoy the best of daily living. Any disorders with your gastrointestinal tract will seriously reduce your powers of assimilation, and this will lower the amount of nutrients reaching your various organs. A healthy digestive system is essential to the enjoyment of a healthy life.

The "burning" sensation you feel, which may be called heartburn, gastritis, dyspepsia or stomach gas, is nature's way of alerting you to upheavals taking place within your gastrointestinal tract. By using easily available power foods, you should be able to cool the burning and restore digestive balance so that food can then be properly metabolized to give your body a much-needed supply of health-building nutrients.

Correct Living Errors and Enjoy Better Digestive Health

Be good to your gastrointestinal tract and it will reward you with better digestive health. Begin by eliminating caffeine-containing irritants such as coffee, tea, cola drinks and chocolate. Switch to Postum, herbal tea, fruit and vegetable drinks. Cut down or eliminate refined sweets and carbohydrates which tend to upset your digestive system and interfere with normal food absorption. Fresh fruits will satisfy your sweet tooth and also provide Vitamin C-sparked energy to alert a sluggish gastrointestinal tract to create better health. Give up smoking and drinking; they burn delicate cells and tissues of your stomach lining (not to mention almost all other parts of your body) and cause destructive injury that is often irreparable. Eat only when relaxed. Drink liquids an hour before or an hour after your meal. Do not overload your digestive system with liquids since this dilutes your enzymatic juices and weakens their powers, giving your disturbances. With these simple corrective measures in daily living, you'll do much to help energize better digestive metabolism.

HOW CARROTS CREATE MIRACLE HEALING AND REJUVENATION OF DIGESTIVE ORGANS

Freshly cooked and eaten carrots become power foods without comparison because they are able to heal and rejuvenate your digestive organs. Carrots are highly concentrated sources of such essential minerals as potassium, magnesium, phosphorus, calcium, sulphur and other trace elements that work to coat the inflamed gastrointestinal components almost within moments. These electrolyte components then "cool" the burning sensation that appears to come from an irritated colon, and restore internal equilibrium.

How to Use This Power Food: Drink carrot juice. You can make it at home with a juice extractor, or you may use canned or bottled carrot juice, available at most supermarkets and health stores. As an alternative, grate raw carrots, flavor with a bit of vegetable oil and a sprinkle of herbs and then eat slowly. You may also slice or dice carrots, steam until tender in a bit of oil, then add some yogurt or a little melted butter; chew thoroughly before swallowing. You may also use chopped or diced carrots as part of a salad with cooked peas or brown rice. If your jaws (and teeth) are strong enough, eat raw carrots. Be sure to chew thoroughly to enable your digestive enzymes to properly metabolize the important minerals that might otherwise be "locked" into the tough fibrous portions of the carrot.

This power food is also a high concentrated source of Vitamin A which is transformed by your intestines into a nutrient that maintains proper gastrointestinal cellular moisture and boosts resistance to infection in this region. The metabolized Vitamin A from carrots is believed to create an antibiotic action within the gastrointestinal tract so that harmful fungus-caused ailments can be healed almost as soon as they begin. This makes carrots a power food that is able to rejuvenate your gastrointestinal tract very speedily.

THE TROPICAL POWER FOOD THAT REVITALIZES YOUR DIGESTIVE SYSTEM

As a luscious tropical fruit, the papaya offers you more than juicy good taste. It offers you a dynamic source of enzymes, known as *papains*, which create miraculous revitalization of the components of your gastrointestinal tract. In particular, the papaya offers you the proteolytic enzymes known as alpha and beta papain and also chymopapain. (Proteolytic enzymes have the power to break down stubborn foods and then extract their healing nutrients which are needed by your gastrointestinal segments.)

The *papain* enzymes also work to metabolize the connective tissues and muscle fibers of meat, drawing out the essential amino acids that are vital to digestive health. These same *papain* enzymes work to break down fatty tissues so that digestion is not only speedier but also more comfortable and effective. With the help of papaya enzymes, there will be a reduced incidence of churning, burning, rumbling and so-called "digestive difficulties" after a main meal.

How to Use This Power Food: Peel and slice and eat fresh papaya either with or after any meal. Use papaya fruit slices for a snack throughout the day. If this fruit is unavailable because it is out of season, use the canned or bottled variety often available in supermarkets and most health stores. Papaya juice is also available at health stores. It is a refreshing, digestion-comforting beverage that you can enjoy after a meal.

THE SPICE THAT COOLS AND REFRESHES YOUR DIGESTIVE SYSTEM

As a power food, the peppermint herb has been used ever since recorded history. The ancient Egyptians, according to hieroglyphics, relied upon peppermint as prescribed by royal court physicians to ease burning, soothe gastritis (inflammation of the stomach lining), comfort dyspepsia (chronic indigestion), ease problems of gas and bloating as we know them today. Today, peppermint tea (from health store or herbal pharmacies) is a spice beverage that will cool and refresh your entire digestive system.

Dissolves Mucus, Cools Tissues, Is Antispasmodic. When you brew the leaves and flowering parts of the peppermint herb, you release astringent substances that tend to dissolve and wash away mucus from your alimentary tract (food tube from throat to intestines). These astringent substances cool inflamed tissues and calm down fluttery muscles by creating an antispasmodic healing. The peppermint astringents also tend to neutralize the strong stomach acid that would ordinarily irritate the esophageal membranes and cause heartburn. With the help of peppermint astringents, the acid is diluted and then washed out before it can cause discomfort.

Free yourself from digestive distress with the help of a cup of freshly brewed peppermint tea after your main meal. Sip it when comfortably hot but *not* scalding.

Suggestion: For a more complete digestive-rejuvenation program, try a combination of these refreshing power foods—fresh papaya fruit as a dessert and then a cup of delicious peppermint tea. You'll have double protection and double healing.

With the help of these tasty power foods, your digestive system should become revitalized and your entire body will look and feel more youthfully healthy through better and more vigorous metabolism.

See Bladder, Colitis, Constipation, Cramps, Diarrhea, Diverticulosis, Nausea, Urinary Problems.

DIVERTICULOSIS
Power foods that protect against bowel "pockets"

Diverticulosis is the presence of small bulges or "pockets" at weak areas of the wall of the colon. It is an ailment of the large bowel (colon) in which the small pouches (diverticula) on its inner surface become packed with wastes, then irritated and inflamed, sometimes causing abscesses. If the infected pockets develop complications of perforation or obstruction, it can become quite serious.

The general course of the ailment starts with abdominal distress, which soon resolves into recurring pain in the lower left region. There may be distention of the abdomen, nausea and complications involving both constipation and diarrhea. If untreated, diverticulosis may cause rectal bleeding which can be a life-threatening condition.

This problem was originally considered an "irritable bowel syndrome," and therapy was aimed at prescribing a low-residue, soft diet. But this food regimen aggravates the condition since, as it later became known, diverticulosis develops *because* of a refined and "chewless" type of diet. Therefore, diverticular sufferers would do well to follow a food program that is high in fiber (roughage or bran) from whole grains, fruits, vegetables, well-chewed seeds and nuts. These are power foods that can help you conquer the problem of bowel pockets.

THE HIGH FIBER WAY TO BOWEL HEALING

High fiber, especially in the form of bran, is a power food way to help heal bowel pockets and related disorders. When you eat bran, the outer coating of the wheat kernel, you send a power food source directly into your digestive-intestinal system. Bran tends to absorb up to ten times its own weight in body liquid and this promotes the passage of bulkier, softer stools. This type of stool is desirable because hard stools form high-pressure segments along the bowel which can cause eruption or bursting of diverticula and this may lead to serious consequences. Therefore, using bran as a power food is helpful in stabilizing intestinal regularity *without* assaulting the delicate pockets.

Swift Healing Action. Bran fiber acts directly on the intestinal microflora, either inhibiting or removing the production of diverticula-causing substances. A most important benefit of this power food is that it hastens the removal of waste from the bowel so that the sensitive intestinal lining is not subjected to prolonged corrosive-erosive attack. The longer waste matter remains in contact with the intestinal lining, the greater is the risk of diverticula formation, along with other irritations.

Consumed regularly, bran will ease pressures on the intestinal lining, protect against pocket formation, and promote swifter healing of irritations already formed.

Increases Moisture, Bulk. Bran fiber is a power food that increases moisture content and bulk of the stool. This dilutes the concentration of potential pocket-forming irritants. Bran fiber thus blocks their contact with the intestinal wall, creating a protective shield or insulation for this organ. The calming, bland, demulcent qualities of this power food help heal the intestinal walls and promote greater protection against the forming of pockets.

How to Use This Power Food: Whole bran is available at all health stores, supermarkets and pharmacies. Sprinkle it over whole grain cereals, both cooked and raw. Add it to soups, stews, casseroles, baked breads, muffins, rolls. Blenderize it with fruit or vegetable juices for a healthful beverage. Plan to use at least six to eight teaspoons of bran daily for greater intestinal health.

Other Power Foods for Digestive-Intestinal Health. Fresh raw fruits and vegetables, well-chewed seeds and nuts, wheat germ, whole grain cereals and breads. Citrus fruits are great fiber sources, but *keep the fibrous membranes* when you peel oranges, grapefruits, tangerines. Chew them along with the pitted fruit pulp for high fiber intake. Try kasha (buckwheat groats), bulgur wheat, couscous. These are delicious whole grain high-fiber power foods available in all supermarkets and health stores. Enjoy brown rice regularly for another good power food. Eat cereals and breads made from oats, rye, whole wheat, triticale (a newly developed grain variety), sesame, sunflower, barley. Cooked beans and peas are other power foods that will give you highly beneficial, intestine-healing fiber and roughage.

With the use of these varieties of power foods, you can enjoy greater intestinal health and freedom from the health risk of diverticulosis.

See Bladder, Colitis, Constipation, Cramps, Diarrhea, Digestive Disturbances, Hemorrhoids.

DIZZINESS
Power foods that restore your body balance

Dizziness (or vertigo) is more than just distressing; it can also be serious. If this condition is accompanied by hypertension, it can break down the entire body. Basically, all cases of dizziness are traced to some disturbance or disorder of the balancing mechanism situated in the inner ear. If there is an accumulation of wax in the ear or a physical injury, dizziness is nature's way of telling you to have these problems corrected.

Dizziness or loss of equilibrium may also be caused by alcohol, salicylates (aspirins and their compounds), medication designed to lower high blood pressure, nicotine from tobacco.

If You Change Position. Some people experience a drop in blood pressure when changing from a recumbent position to an erect one, and this can cause a transient giddiness. It can also occur in older folks if there is a sudden head movement, especially when looking upwards. To help guard against dizziness, do not make such swift position changes. Take a moment to mentally and physically prepare yourself, then do so gently. This will help protect you against these symptoms.

Low Blood Sugar Correction Helps Overcome Dizziness. To protect yourself against dizziness, you need to maintain a balanced blood sugar level. In particular, you need glucose, a natural blood sugar that nourishes your brain which is then able to send forth instant messages to your body to maintain balanced posture. A normal glucose level in the blood is maintained at a fairly constant range (between 60 to 100 milligrams per 100 milliliters of blood). If it falls below this range, you may experience weakness, shaking, blurred vision and dizziness. To help correct this form of dizziness, a power food program is aimed at helping to increase the blood glucose levels so that the bloodstream will be able to supply nourishment to the brain at a steady level.

Power Food Program to Protect Against Dizziness. Begin by eliminating all man-made sugar products. All processed foods containing sugar in any form should be eliminated. Read labels of packaged foods. If in doubt, don't use the product. Do not use sugar from a shaker or in cooking. Eliminate caffeine-containing beverages such as coffee, tea, cola or soda. Use such dizziness-preventing power foods as lean meats, fish, eggs, dairy products, seeds, beans, nuts, fresh fruits and vegetables and their juices. Herb teas, Postum, chemical-free club sodas are other helpful power foods. Most of them are prime sources of power-packed protein, vitamins, minerals, *natural* carbohydrates which work swiftly to raise your glucose levels and send a supply of energy to your brain cells to protect against weakness that could lead to dizziness.

Power Food Dizziness-Control Beverage. Although she is only in her middle 50's, Adele Z. started to become dizzy and fall, much like a person much older. Adele Z. had no organic ailments, yet she frequently had the "shakes," intense irritability and a few blackouts. When she lost self-control on a public street and fainted, she was rushed to a local health center. Here it was noted that she needed a special power food that would raise her too-low glucose levels so that her starved brain cells could be adequately nourished. That power food was *protein.* But more important, the protein had to be energized swiftly so it could be used within a matter of moments by the sluggish brain cells that were responsible for her vertigo. So this *Power Food Dizziness-Control Beverage* was created for Adele Z. She drinks it every morning. No longer is she dizzy. Her hands are steady, she is cheerful, and blackouts have dimmed in her memory and no longer recur. Here is the power food beverage:

1 teaspoon brewer's yeast powder
2 tablespoons honey
½ cup orange juice
1 tablespoon lecithin granules
½ cup skim milk

Blenderize for a moment or stir vigorously until all items are assimilated. Drink slowly. Drink just one glass a day for a surge of youthful vitality that has a double benefit: you will be energized from head to toe, and you will no longer feel dizzy.

Works Swiftly, Effectively, Is Longer-Lasting. The protein from the skim milk combines with the B-complex of the brewer's yeast and protein from the lecithin. It is energized by the concentrated Vitamin C from the orange juice and the natural concentrated carbohydrates of the honey. In this form, it is almost instantly absorbed by the bloodstream, and sent shooting upward to the brain for swift, effective and longer-lasting production of vitality. Your well-energized brain is now able to help you walk and think and talk without the threat of dizziness.

Grapes and Grape Juice: Power Foods That Conquer Dizziness. A handful of grapes that can be eaten anywhere—while standing on line, while commuting, while walking, while in a building, while at work or recreation—will help conquer dizziness. Here is a power food that is a high concentration of fructose that provides speedy, almost instant brain and body energy. Grape juice too is a power food that acts like a whiff of smelling salts—but it is a natural stimulant. Just drink a glass of grape juice daily for a powerful brain and body balance booster.

Benefits: This power food, either eaten whole or juiced, causes an immediate release of stored glycogen from the liver to be dispersed through the central nervous system via the bloodstream, upward to the brain. Here, the parched or dehydrated brain cells are nourished with the fructose to make you feel immediately alert and awake. Your dizzy feeling subsides almost as quickly as it came on.

Suggestion: Carry grapes for snacks to build resistance to dizziness. Also, carry a packet of sun-dried raisins (grapes without water) because they are high-power concentrates of fructose that act with dynamic swiftness in giving you good balance, clear thinking, alert senses.

With these tasty, refreshing power food beverages and foods, you should be able to enjoy a life without dizziness and with much better health.

See Fainting, Fatigue, Low Blood Sugar, Trembling, Weakness.

EARS
Power foods that prevent or soothe earaches

Your ear serves the purpose of hearing—but also the vital function of maintaining body equilibrium. If you lose only partial hearing, you tend to become unbalanced in your walking, your talking, even your vision. While such symptoms may not be too noticeable, they do tend to force you into an off-centered equilibrium. You may have to turn your head to hear words in your "good" ear. You find it necessary to lean to one side or the other since you are better able to hear that way.

Sound waves strike your eardrum (tympanic membrane) making it vibrate, and therefore you hear. But when you have an earache, there is a muffling of these impulses and the acoustic nerve in your brain cannot transmit them. You feel inadequate as you try to make both your ears do the work that only one is capable of doing. This creates a form of tension that may result in earaches and other disorders.

Protect Against These Earache Causes. Repeated loud noises can cause earache. A blow to the ear can injure an acoustic nerve and bring about aches as well as possible hearing loss. Certain medications may destroy the delicate cells of the hearing apparatus; these would include quinine, streptomycin, gentamicin, some antibiotics. They cause possible destruction of the acoustic nerve components and bring on earache together with hearing loss. Arsenic, mercury and overindulgence in alcohol and tobacco may cause a blockage of the arteries so that the acoustic nerve is starved because insufficient nutrient-carrying blood reaches the acoustic nerve.

Vegetable Oils as Earache Healers. To open up blocked arteries so that they can transport essential nutrients to your acoustic components, switch to the use of vegetable oils. These are power foods that should replace hard fats such as butter and even margarine. Cut down or eliminate intake of animal fat foods. The potent polyunsaturates and essential fatty acids in vegetable oils have an emulsifying power in that they can help melt and dissolve accumulations that are choking the arteries near your auditory canal and preventing transport of important nutrition. Vegetable oils are power foods that unblock and then lubricate the auditory-acoustic nerves so that they are "washed" and able to respond to external stimuli. Just one week on this low hard fat program and increased vegetable oil power food program should help re-establish better hearing and freedom from earaches.

Power Food Earache Healer. Boil one garlic clove in one-half cup of water until soft but not mushy. Place the cooled garlic clove on the outside of the ear but *do NOT push it down the ear canal!* Cover with a bit of clean cotton. Keep in place with adhesive tape. Let remain all day (replace daily with new boiled clove) until the earache infection is drawn out.

Benefit: Volatile antiseptic ingredients in the garlic will seek out, nullify, cleanse and draw out infectious causes of the ache.

Garlic Oil Power Food. Place or drop warm (not hot) garlic oil in each ear to clear out and detoxify infections, and then ease and eliminate the ache. Healing occurs after just two or three such once-a-day power food applications.

Yogurt + Wheat Germ = Earache Healer. In a cup of plain skim milk yogurt, stir two tablespoons of wheat germ. Eat slowly. Three cups in one day should help soothe and comfort the ear segments and ease the ache.

Benefit: The yogurt is a source of highly concentrated calcium, a soothing mineral that combines with the powerful B-complex vitamins in the wheat germ. Together, they work to soothe the acoustic and auditory nerves of the ear which are irritated and aching. The calcium pampers the nerves while the B-complex works to replenish any frazzled or jagged cellular destruction wrought by noise pollution. This form of reparation will bring about a power healing within a day, at the most. By soothing the central nervous system at the same time, this power food combo is able to help ease many other body aches.

Power Food Ache-Healing Tonic. In one glass of any vegetable juice, add two tablespoons of lecithin granules (from health store or pharmacy). Stir or blenderize. Drink two or three glasses of this *Power Food Ache-Healing Tonic* during the day. Your earache will be soothed within hours after taking. Often, just one glass will help create this most welcome healing.

Benefit: Derived from soybeans, lecithin is a powerhouse source of choline, a substance that is able to penetrate the blood-brain barrier, then stimulate the brain cells to produce more acetylcholine, a substance that can transmit "locked" nerve impulses. As a consequence, the congestion is eased and the ache is relieved.

Free your ears (and body) of recurring aches with the help of these quick-to-prepare, healing power foods and beverages.

See Dizziness, Hearing Problems.

EMPHYSEMA
Power foods that oxygenate your breathing apparatus

Breathing becomes impaired when the lungs start to lose their youthful elasticity, causing them to be continuously overdistended. This condition is known as *emphysema.* The word is derived from the Greek, meaning "bodily inflation." It refers to a condition characterized by air-filled expansion of lung tissues. As a result, not enough air can move freely in and out of your lungs. While you are usually able to breath *in*, it is difficult to breathe *out*. Your lungs are in a constant state of inflation.

Symptoms, Complications. Shortness of breath on exertion is the earliest symptom. There may be a hard cough which causes fatigue. After talking or laughter, a hacking cough seizes hold and causes various amounts of chest pain. As exhaling becomes more difficult, the chest takes on a barrel-like appearance. Between inhaling and exhaling, you may need to pause. In more advanced cases, there may be a condition of cyanosis. (This is a blue appearance of the skin, especially on the face and extremities, indicating a lack of sufficient oxygen in the arterial blood.) If untreated, emphysema becomes more complicated. Breathing apparatus becomes degenerated. There is total body weakness. A more serious complication is that of right heart failure; that is, failure due to venous and capillary engorgement.

Basic Lung Healing Program: Eliminate smoking. Avoid areas that are smoke filled. Avoid pollution. Eliminate abuses to the components of your breathing apparatus. That is, foods and beverages should be neither too hot nor too cold. Avoid lung-irritating harsh seasonings such as salt, pepper, ketchup, mustard, vinegar. For flavorings, use modest amounts of natural herbs and spices. Avoid sudden temperature changes. If you have to go from a hot room into the cold outdoors, or vice versa, hold a clean handkerchief over your nose and mouth. This helps to warm the air going into your respiratory system and avoids causing shock. If it is chilly outdoors, wear a flannel scarf to warm your throat. To help oxygenate your breathing apparatus, be good to your respiratory organs at all times.

HOW TO BREATHE BETTER WITH A POWER FOOD INHALANT

A folklore power food to help reconstruct damaged lung tissue and promote a freer exchange of formerly "locked" air is found in *blue violet leaves.* This sweetly scented medicinal herb from the fields (available at most health stores and herbal pharmacies) contains microscopic but highly concentrated amounts of natural decongestants which unlock the blockage so that you can breathe out and remove accumulated air. When you *inhale* this power food, you open up clogged channels and promote a better exchange of air.

Lung-Cleansing Inhalant: In one cup of freshly boiled water, steep one teaspoon of blue violet leaves for three to four minutes. Put a towel over your head in a tent-like fashion. Now breathe in the fragrance of this *Lung-Cleansing Inhalant.* Do it slowly. Hold your breath for 30 seconds. This enables the herbal decongestants to help unblock the stored-up blockage and promote improved oxygen exchange. Now, breathe out. Keep doing this simple program until the brew has cooled. Discard. Plan to remain indoors for a few hours so your lungs can be healthfully oxygenated without being abused by outdoor pollution and climate. Prepare a fresh *Lung-Cleansing Inhalant* of blue violet leaves at least three times a day. You should be able to enjoy better oxygenation within four to five days. Afterwards, use this simple power food inhalant at least once daily to help protect against further emphysema tissue degeneration.

"BETTER BREATHING POWER TONIC"

Climbing up short staircases left Peter X. feeling breathless. At times, he had such a hacking cough that he had to sit down and try to catch his breath while his face turned all shades of red and blue as the spasms racked his body. Exhaling was a chore. Peter X. brought his problems to a local orthomolecular physician (specialist in nutritional healing) who suggested that he prepare a simple "Better Breathing Power Tonic" to be taken at least three times daily. Peter X. followed this simple advice. Within nine days, he began to breathe better. His stubborn cough just "went away." Now he could climb up staircases with the ease of a youngster. He had used nutrition to help correct his respiratory distress.

How to Prepare "Better Breathing Tonic": To a glass of grapefruit or orange juice, add two tablespoons of wheat germ oil. If possible, blenderize to thoroughly combine the ingredients. Now drink slowly. Plan to drink three glasses daily.

Oxygenation Benefit: The citrus fruit juice is a powerhouse of highly concentrated Vitamin C. This is combined with the Vitamin E of the wheat germ oil in a form that helps inhibit damage to the membranes of the lungs and aid in their reconstruction. A *bonus benefit* is that in this combination, the nutrients appear to ease constrictions and spasms of the smooth muscles of the bronchial tubes. This helps to act as a bulwark against encroaching disorders of emphysema. This "Better Breathing Tonic" is a power food that works speedily and effectively for improved respiratory health.

The Balloon Method for Better Breathing

Improved oxygenation is possible when nutrients are able to penetrate barriers to help repair the damage caused by emphysema. The *Balloon Method* is a simple exercise that enhances the effectiveness of the nutrients in the "Better Breathing Tonic." It helps to control and ease the ravages of emphysema. Here's how to use it:

You need a thick balloon, which will make you red in the face to blow up. Just blow it up until it reaches its capacity. (A very large balloon is more effective and helpful.) Plan to blow up the balloon at least fifteen minutes a day. As soon as the balloon is filled up with air, release it, and start all over again. Just schedule the fifteen-minutes-per-day session.

Benefit: When you keep breathing out, your face shows some exertion. This helps boost a better in-and-out exchange of oxygen within your respiratory system. It unblocks "choked" air and counteracts the ravages of encroaching emphysema. It helps to energize and activate the components of the "Better Breathing Tonic" so that they help promote lung capillary integrity and prevent permeability, a factor involved in emphysema.

With the use of power foods (oxygen is a potent lung food), you will help oxygenate your breathing apparatus and be able to protect yourself against emphysema.

See BREATHING DIFFICULTIES, COUGHS.

EYES
Power foods that heal and strengthen organs of sight

The eye is an amazing feat of human engineering. It is an instantly self-adjusting camera, complete with its own repair system as well as a built-in drainage mechanism to provide adequate moisture for daily use. With proper care and the use of nourishing power foods, the eye should serve you well for your lifetime. In modern times, the eye is often abused by excessive television watching, the erosion of pollution, continuous eyestrain in work, at home and even during recreation. By helping to strengthen the organs of sight, you should be able to heal the cause of insufficient vision.

A Power Food Program for Glaucoma Relief

Problem: There is an increase in pressure within the eye that may cause damage to the optic nerve. No warning symptoms appear early in the ailment. Later, there may be halos or rainbows around electric lights, blind spots, narrowing of the visual field and extremely poor night vision.

Power Food Healing Program: You need to induce natural drainage that has become blocked and is responsible for this internal visual pressure. Eliminate the use of caffeine-containing foods such as coffee, tea, some chocolates, soda pop drinks. These tend to cause blood vessel constriction involved in glaucoma. Eliminate alcohol and tobacco because they restrict free fluid exchange and build up visual pressure. Switch to fresh fruit and vegetable juices. In particular, plan to increase intake of B-complex and calcium foods. These nutrients appear to relieve the intraocular stress condition and promote a freer exchange of fluids.

Suggestion: In a cup of plain yogurt, stir two tablespoons of wheat germ or bran. Eat two or three cups daily. The calcium in the yogurt is energized by the natural carbohydrate B-complex action of the grains to help soothe the taut optical nerves and enable nutrients to pass freely to all portions of your organs of sight.

Say "No" to Salt, Say "Yes" to Lemon Juice. Eliminate salt from cooking and at the table. Avoid any processed foods that contain salt. Instead, flavor with lemon juice.

Benefit: Salt tends to constrict capillaries within the organs of sight and this "chokes" off moisture. It is involved in formation of glaucoma. Lemon juice is a taste-satisfying salt substitute that is also high in catalytic enzymes as well as Vitamin C that will help repair cells and tissues of your visual organs, and help unblock accumulated moisture that may lead to glaucoma. It's the tasty power food way to help improve your vision.

Cataract Relief with Power Foods

Problem: There is a slowly increasing opaqueness in the eye lens. Diminishing vision is gradual. In more advanced situations, it is like a window frosted by the cold and only a much-shaded light can be seen through it.

Power Food Healing Program: Boost your intake of these three groups of power foods:

1. *Protein.* Lean meat, fish, eggs, dairy products, peas, beans, seeds, nuts. *Cataract Relief Benefit:* This problem is often traced to a protein deficiency. Healthy eye lenses contain about 35% soluble protein; but lenses showing cataract opacification contain decreasing amounts of soluble protein and increasing amounts of insoluble protein which appears

to create visual congestion. There is a shifting balance of normal soluble-insoluble protein in the lens, with much protein being lost. This indicates a need for protein intake. *Power Food Suggestion:* To a glass of tomato juice, add one tablespoon of brewer's yeast. Stir or blenderize. Drink slowly. This is a powerhouse of concentrated soluble protein needed to help ease risk of cataract development. Drink at least three glasses daily.

2. *Vitamin C.* All citrus fruits and their juices, tomatoes, pineapples, broccoli, green pepper, cabbage, cauliflower, potatoes. *Cataract Relief Benefit:* Vitamin C in these foods is needed to replace that which appears to dry out in the eye lens in certain forms of cataract. The aqueous humor and lens need a high concentration of Vitamin C to help absorb the opacity and offer hope for better vision. *Power Food Suggestion:* Eat raw fruit salads daily. Drink fruit juices throughout the day. Have a raw vegetable salad with steamed potatoes for another power-packed source of sight-saving Vitamin C.

3. *Vitamin D.* Milk, butter, egg yolk, herring, salmon, tuna, fish liver oils. *Cataract Relief Benefit:* This vitamin is able to better metabolize calcium and thereby provide important nourishment for the sight organs. Vitamin D acts upon calcium to help prevent zonular cataract, a form that is most prevalent. *Power Food Suggestion:* A salmon or tuna salad regularly is beneficial. In a glass of milk (use skim milk if fat or calorie watching), put one tablespoon of cod liver oil. Stir or blenderize. Drink slowly. The calcium of the milk combines with the Vitamin D of the oil to help restore nutritive balance and protection against cataract in the eye lens.

Power Food Programs to Boost Visual Strength

Visual disorders such as astigmatism (blurred vision), near and far sightedness, presbyopia (middle-aged sight), may respond to the invigoration offered by power food programs.

First Step: You must eliminate use of alcohol and tobacco. These narcotics cause eye muscle palsies that injure the nerves leading to the eye muscles. Vision weakness and deterioration then take place. Quit these bad habits and your eyes (as well as your body) will become much healthier and younger looking, too.

Eat Citrus Fruits with White Rind. The white, thread-like covering on oranges, grapefruits, tangerines are powerhouses of highly concentrated bioflavonoids. When you peel these citrus fruits, plan to eat the fruit *with* these threads. You introduce a high concentration of bioflavonoids which are needed to nourish capillaries involved in better vision.

Eye-Nourishing Tonic: Pour one quart of boiled water over one cup of fresh parsley. Let steep for 20 minutes. Strain and drink at least three cups daily. You have a powerhouse of vitamins that are helpful for the rods and cones of your retina and eye muscles.

Eye-Soothing Poultice. Here's a power food you use externally. Grate a raw scrubbed potato and use as a poultice on your closed eyes for 20 minutes. Rinse with warm and then cool water. The Vitamin C, potassium and phosphorus combine to nourish irritated membranes, repair visual tissues, and improve the strength of your eyes.

Blurred, Indistinct Vision. Scrape or grate a raw washed apple and use as a poultice on your closed eyes for 20 minutes. Afterward wash off with contrasting warm and cool water.

Benefit: The high pectin-hemicellulose content together with Vitamins A and C of the apple will help draw out the toxins responsible for swelling visual membranes. This will soothe irritation. Vision will be less blurred and more distinct. Try this power food poultice once a day.

With the use of power foods and improved health care, you can help refresh and rejuvenate your eyes.

See HEADACHES.

FAINTING
Power foods that prevent and eliminate fainting

Fainting is usually a problem affecting people who have to stand for long, unrelieved periods of time. Fainting may also occur when you are subjected to high, humid temperature, insufficient sleep, excessive physical and/or mental work, poorly ventilated rooms and even an abrupt altitude change, either going up or coming down!

You can anticipate a fainting spell if there is a feeling of oppression in the heart. There may be a too-fast heartbeat, very swift and deep breathing. The fingers and toes feel numb or cold, or both. There may be other symptoms such as dizziness, dim vision, shaking and sweating. Women tend to faint more readily than men. Often, fainting may be traced to the body's reaction to drugs which lower blood pressure, an insulin overdosage, even headache preparations.

If you notice a faint feeling after any of these things, correct these errors and you should be able to prevent and eliminate fainting.

THE MORNING POWER FOOD FOR DAY-LONG FREEDOM FROM FAINTING

Honey is a sweet power food that can stimulate your sluggish responses and provide tasty protection against the problem of fainting. It is an especially beneficial food if taken in the morning.

Because honey is an inverted and highly concentrated natural sugar, it does not ferment in the digestive system; it remains there, and in a "time release" action will help raise your blood sugar levels at a steady rate in balance with your activities. If you take several spoons of honey in the morning, spread upon a thick slice of whole grain bread, or stirred into a cup of herbal tea or coffee substitute such as Postum, you'll be supercharging your sluggish system to give you day-long vitality and freedom from fainting. It's the sweet power food you will love to take.

POWER FOOD SANDWICH FOR ELIMINATION OF FAINTING

A concentrated form of protein will help correct the blood sugar imbalance responsible for that faint feeling. A unique benefit of a special power food is that it is so supercharged with protein and many of the essential amino acids that if you eat this food as a sandwich earlier in the day or at lunchtime, you will be revitalizing your sluggish bloodstream so that more oxygen can be dispersed to your brain cells, thereby eliminating the risk of fainting. It works within minutes, too!

Power Food Sandwich. Natural peanut butter without salt, spread on thick slices of whole grain bread, together with fruit puree (instead of sugar jam) gives your body an "instant" reaction so that the elevated blood sugar eliminates any tendency to faint. Eat this sandwich, together with a glass of orange or grapefruit juice, and you'll revitalize your entire system.

Benefits: Natural peanut butter is a dynamic source of protein together with phosphorus and potassium. In this combo, the protein is literally "shot forth" by the electrifying vigor of the two minerals and sent surging through your bloodstream to wake up your tired cells. This helps nourish your brain cells and the fainting urge is blocked and then eliminated. Plan to eat this *Power Food Sandwich* at least once daily to help give you natural resistance against fainting.

Power Food Inhalant. Grate a raw horseradish or, better yet, carry a small bottle of prepared horseradish, available in all supermarkets. If you should feel a fainting spell, just inhale briefly of this horseradish. In a moment, the fainting feeling is gone and you now feel more vigorous and alert.

Wake up your sluggish system so that you will be energetic under most circumstances. Use power foods that will help give you preventive immunity and elimination of this unpleasant condition.

See Dizziness, Fatigue, Low Blood Sugar, Mental Alertness, Weakness.

FATIGUE (TIREDNESS)
Power foods that recharge your energy sites

What makes you feel tired so much of the time? The key to unlocking this mystery lies in a component situated within your brain. Called the *hypothalamus*, this is an endocrine gland involved in the functions of the autonomic nervous system.

Body and mind energy is ruled by the activity of the hypothalamus. If it is well nourished with an adequate supply of glucose (body sugar), it sends forth transmitting signals to help you keep energetic both physically and mentally. But if your hypothalamus is deficient in the important nutrients of natural carbohydrates and (most important) protein, it functions erratically. This may lead to fatigue and that feeling of being tired all too often. In many situations, it may cause premature aging. Some people let this tiredness get the best of them and shuffle along with a stooped gait, bleary eyes and a depletion of normal energy. With correction of the "starved" hypothalamus, you can help recharge your energy sites to wipe away fatigue and make you feel youthfully energetic.

THE POWER FOOD SNACK THAT DOUBLES ENERGY IN MINUTES

Gladys G. felt youthful energy slipping through her fingers. She began to look haggard and wan. Driving her car for a few blocks became terrifying because she had slow reflexes and could not manage quick signals. She had a part-time job (which was threatened because of her loss of energy) together with household duties (which were neglected because all she wanted to do was lie in bed or slump on the couch). Gladys G. was in her early 50's but looked and felt in her 90's, as she lamented!

Sunflower Seeds—a Quick Way to Energy. A jogging neighbor heard her complaint and shared her secret of unlimited energy. In addition to daily jogging, the ever-energetic neighbor was able to hold down a fulltime job and manage a busy household. What was her secret? The neighbor liked to snack—on sunflower seeds! The high-vitality-filled neighbor would carry a bag of shelled sunflower seeds with her and snack on them throughout the day. This was her secret power food. She told Gladys G. to snack on seeds early in the morning and whenever she felt a letdown. Gladys G. tried it. Within minutes, her weakness vanished. She felt alert, active and alive again! She looked brighter within two days. She could drive in busy traffic with youthful reflexes. Now she just breezed through her job and household tasks. She even started jogging as a means of using up her "energy surplus," as she called it!

Benefits. A powerhouse of highly concentrated protein, the seeds send a supercharged energy through your circulatory system, then to your brain cells to nourish the source of vitality: your hypothalamus. Protein is seized by your metabolic processes and transformed into essential amino acids that then release a steady supply of glucose. This provides oxygenated nourishment for your hypothalamus. But a super benefit here is that there is an *immediate* as well as *steady* release of amino-acid-created glucose to your hypothalamus. Therefore, eating this power food will give your hypothalamus a time release benefit for day-long energy.

Simple Program: Carry a bag of sunflower seeds with you at all times. *Power Benefits:* Munch a handful or two whenever you feel fatigue or any form of tiredness. Within a few moments, your glucose-invigorated hypothalamus will wipe away fatigue and fill you with youthful energy. Sunflower seeds are power food snacks that taste every bit as good as they make you feel!

THE SWEET POWER FOOD THAT ACTIVATES YOUR ENERGY SITES—IN A HURRY

Need a quick lift? Want to activate your energy sites in a hurry? Try this sweet power food—*raisins*.

As a sun-dried power food, raisins contain the naturally sweet grape sugar in a highly concentrated form. When you eat a handful of raisins, the glucose is speedily metabolized without the need of much insulin. This glucose is sent almost immediately to your brain cells for hypothalamus stimulation. It creates almost instant energy to help make you feel alert and active in a hurry.

The hydrogen ion concentration of raisin glucose will combine with the amino acids in your body to promote this brain-stimulating action to help recharge your energy sites almost immediately.

Simple Program: Carry a small package of sun-dried raisins with you Do *not* use raisins that have been treated with sulphur dioxide or any other chemical since this can cause cell-tissue upheaval. Read package labels. Health stores have sun-dried raisins, properly designed. Eat a handful. You'll get a natural lift in a hurry. You'll feel alert and active in body and mind as your energy sites send forth youthful vitality.

Free your body from fatigue and tiredness with the use of these delicious power foods that are every bit as good as the youthful energy they provide.

See Dizziness, Fainting, Low Blood Sugar, Mental Alertness, Weakness.

FEVER
Power foods that cool and soothe excessive body heat

A fever is a condition in which your body temperature has risen too high. Basically, it is an early-warning signal that something has gone amiss with your body and corrective measures should be taken.

A normal temperature is one that falls in a range between 97°F. and 99°F.

Your temperature undergoes frequent changes during the day. It rises during late afternoon or early evening. It is likely to be a little higher after meals. Strong exertion or heavy exercise will also cause a temperature rise. If your body temperature is elevated beyond a reasonable daily variation, then this body heat is in need of cooling off with the use of power foods.

FRUIT AND VEGETABLE FASTING PROGRAM FOR FEVER RELIEF

For one day, plan a fruit and vegetable fast. Eat and drink nothing else but fresh raw fruits and vegetables and their juices. The high-powered mineral content of these plant foods will help detoxify your system, influence your brain's thermostat and regulate it so that you will soon feel cool all over.

Benefits of High Power Fasting Program: A fever usually causes electrolytes (minerals) to become burned up at a rapid rate. This causes depletion. At the same time, a fever lowers your body's resistance to harmful bacteria. These enter your bloodstream, flow up to the base of your brain to threaten a group of sensitively gathered cells. Alarmed by the poisons, the cells need mineral invigoration to send emergency methods to your other body parts to help regulate heat balance. Without these minerals, the cells cannot transmit the messages and the fever intensifies. With the availability of fruit and vegetable minerals, the cells become strong and are able to create a vascular balance so that the heating mechanism is better balanced. When your body is able to metabolize minerals without interference of other nutrients (such as during a fast), then it is better able to cope with and correct feverish conditions.

During a fruit and vegetable fasting program, germ-damaged body cells are rapidly flushed out to make room for healthy new cell replacements. The minerals from these power foods alert your brain's thermostat to send forth emergency signals to regulate the heart beat, stabilize the rate of breathing and adjust the flow of blood through arteries and veins. Just one day on this fruit and vegetable fasting program can do much to cool and soothe excessive body heat.

Power Food Juices Cool Off Fever. Whenever Allan L. feels a fever coming on, he follows the advice given to him by a physical training specialist. He prepares some simple Power Food Juices, using peeled cucumbers, lettuce, carrots, celery (either singly or in any desired combination), and drinks two or three or even four glasses daily. Within a few hours, Allan L.'s fever is gone. He is cooled and healed.

Benefits: Raw vegetable juices are prime sources of such minerals as potassium, phosphorus and iron which are needed to maintain a better body water balance. These minerals are immediately absorbed by the bloodstream and then sent to the brain cells to wash them free of heat-causing toxins and thereby cool off the entire body. With the use of these Power Food Juices, you can actually drink away your fever!

Cool Off with a Water Soak. Immerse yourself in a tub of comfortably cool water, a power "food" that is healing both internally and externally. Help yourself to cool off by placing an ice bag on your head. The benefit here is that the ice will cool off your constricted scalp arteries, so that there can be a better blood flow to the rest of your body, which is cooled off in the water. In effect, this water soak "washes out" the fever-causing toxins from your head and the rest of your body. A 20-minute water soak is a pleasant and effective way to help cool and soothe excessive body heat.

Alcohol-Water Sponge. Another way to cool off a fever is to sponge the skin with a combination of alcohol and water. The process of evaporation requires heat. This external power healer draws the heat to the surface and casts it out, thereby reducing body temperature. It is a natural antipyretic or fever-healer.

Fever-Cooling Power Potion. In a glass of any desired vegetable juice, stir two tablespoons of a high-protein powder (from health store or pharmacy) and one tablespoon of brewer's yeast powder. Stir or blenderize vigorously. Drink three glasses daily. Your fever should subside almost by nightfall.

Benefit: Fever increases the metabolic rate and therefore increases oxygen demand. The higher the fever, the higher the oxygen demand which your body may not be able to supply. Meet this requirement with the *Fever-Cooling Power Potion*. The electrolyte minerals of the juice seize hold of the quickly prepared amino acids of the protein powder, and become energized by the B-complex vitamins of the brewer's yeast. This *triple-power* action stabilizes your runaway metabolism, restores normalcy, and at the same time will meet oxygen demands (via B-complex action) and also regulate this level. Within a few hours, several glasses of this *Fever-Cooling Power Potion* will restore soothing balance so you'll feel good again. You will have conquered the fever with power foods!

With the help of everyday power foods, you should be able to tame that runaway fever, and cool and soothe your excessively heated body quickly.

See COLDS, FATIGUE, LOW BLOOD SUGAR, TREMBLING, WEAKNESS.

FOOT PROBLEMS
Power foods that heal and strengthen your feet

When your feet hurt, your body hurts all over. Besides the usual foot ailments, such seemingly unrelated complaints as bachache, headaches, fatigue and irritability can often be traced down to your feet, the barometer for your body's overall health.

With proper care, your feet can serve you well so that you will be able to walk, stand, perform daily activities with youthful energy and vigor.

Power foods are able to improve your circulation, smooth out rough skin blemishes and strengthen your bones (52 in both feet) so that your ligaments (214 in both feet) will be flexible and powerful with the forward locomotion vigor of a young person.

Begin with Better Foot Posture. To heal and strengthen your feet, begin by observing the basic laws of better posture. You need to learn to stand and walk with your feet parallel. When you take a step forward, put your body weight *first* on your heel. As you go forward, transfer weight to your outer arch, then across the ball of your foot and finally to your big toe. Repeat this rhythmic process as you continue walking. Many of your foot (and body) ills could be prevented with this simple foot posture program.

Better Arch Support = Freedom from Foot Pain. Whether standing or walking, adjust your posture so that you put your body weight on the *outside* arch of your foot, which is made of bone for the specific purpose of bearing this weight. This creates a *natural* arch support that will help free you from foot (and body) pain. *Caution:* When you stand or walk incorrectly with an improper posture, your body weight is forced into the *inside* arch of your foot, causing severe strain. Your bones, ligaments and muscles eventually give way to the pressure and this causes "fallen arches," leading not only to severe foot pain, but also to related leg, pelvis, back, neck and head pains. So learn to put more or all pressure on your *outside* arch to help make you walk better and feel better all over.

THE POWER FOOD THAT PROMOTES YOUTHFUL FOOT CIRCULATION

Troubled with aching calf muscles as well as sudden painful spasms in the soles of her feet, Norma O'B. felt like an invalid. She was often confined to her chair because of the shooting spasms of pain from her soles right up to her knees. Norma O'B. told her podiatrist about her problems and he recommended a simple power food that would help dissolve the accumulated debris that was causing venous-arterial congestion in her lower extremities. That power food was *wheat germ oil*. Norma O'B. was advised to take at least 750 units daily. (Supplements are available in health stores and pharmacies.) She took the power food, and within nine days her calf and foot muscles felt more resilient. She was soon able to walk, stand and run, too, because her legs felt youthful again.

Benefits: Wheat germ oil, whether in capsules or as a free-flowing oil for use as a salad dressing or in cooking, is a highly concentrated source of Vitamin E. This nutrient is able to unblock congestion of the veins and arteries involved in better foot health. It sends a stream of cleansing and nourishing oxygen to the nutrient-starved ligaments and tissues involved in foot flexibility so that your lower limbs and the rest of your body respond with better agility. It is a foot-energizing power food!

HOW TO WARM UP COLD FEET WITH A POWER POWDER

Sprinkle a small amount of cayenne pepper into your shoes to help stimulate your sluggish foot circulation. In a little while, as you walk around, this power powder will warm up your cold feet and help you feel glowing and alive all over.

THE POWER FRUIT THAT REFRESHES TIRED FEET

This golden power fruit, the lemon, contains a treasure of Vitamin C and fructose that appear to refresh and energize the most tired of feet, so that you feel much stronger throughout your body. Try these two methods: (1) Rub a wedge of fresh lemon on the skin of your feet to give you refreshing, tingly relief from tiredness. (2) Soak your feet in a mixture of hot water and the juice of one whole lemon. Rinse in warm water and dry carefully. You'll feel refreshed in a matter of minutes. A bonus benefit is that the lemon juice will whiten the skin of your feet and soften hardness while it soothes.

POWER FOOD COMBO FOR SPARKLING FEET

Mix enough ordinary table salt with olive oil until you have a paste. Now just rub this paste all over your feet. Rub it between your toes, on your soles, on the instep, heels and everywhere else. After 15 minutes, splash off with warm and then comfortably cool water. Your feet will sparkle with youthful agility. In paste form, these two power foods create a form of friction-lubrication reaction that alerts and activates your circulation, making you feel better all over!

POWER FOOD FOR FOOT HEALTH: FROM MILLION-DOLLAR SPA

At a fabulously expensive million-dollar health spa, the tired and aching feet of patrons are treated with a "secret" power food that causes total revitalization of feet and bodies, too. This "secret" power food is the avocado! It works miracles in foot rejuvenation. Now, for the cost of about 50¢, you can give yourself this same million-dollar power food treatment right at home. Here's how:

Mash the pulp of a ripe avocado to a thick puree. To this, add the juice of half a lemon and a tablespoon of vegetable oil. Blend well. Now rub well into your toes, soles, heels and every part of your feet, right up to your ankles. Now put on a pair of clean white socks. Let remain overnight. Next morning, wash thoroughly under contrasting warm and then cool water. Use a rough washcloth. You'll be able to loosen decaying cells and tissues, and wash away debris. You'll soon have very soft and smooth foot skin. More important, your feet will have that "glad to be alive" feeling. Try this million-dollar health spa "secret" power food program for three nights. You'll soon feel as if you're walking on air!

Give new power to your feet with the help of these various power foods. You'll feel youthfully happy all over.

See Gout, Leg and Foot Problems, Stiffness, Varicose Veins.

GALLBLADDER
Power foods that protect against gallstones and improve gallbladder function

Your gallbladder is a pear-shaped pouch on the underside of your liver. Its purpose is to store and concentrate bile, which comes from your liver through a special duct to be delivered to the intestines via another duct. As a bile-storage organ, your gallbladder is needed to help you digest fat, an important nutrient needed by all parts of your body. If your gallbladder does not properly function, it sets off a chain reaction of other health problems that may lead to body aging and gallstones, too.

Symptoms: An unhealthy gallbladder may give you gaseous indigestion, irregularity, visual disturbances, poor fat digestion, bloating, and skin lesions—because fat is improperly absorbed. In more serious gallbladder malfunction, the skin turns pasty white or yellowish; the eyes may also become discolored. Stones may be formed in the common bile duct. This obstruction may cause infection along with jaundice and liver injury. If a gallbladder attack results from a stone in the bile duct, there are severe pains radiating from the upper abdomen to the back or right shoulder.

With proper health care and the use of power foods, you should be able to enjoy a healthy gallbladder and freedom from the risk of gallstones.

THE POWER FOOD THAT LUBRICATES YOUR GALLBLADDER

Simple olive oil is a miraculous power food that can wake up a sleepy gallbladder and lubricate its components and ducts, so that it can store and then release bile as needed to metabolize needed Vitamins A, D, E and K which *must* have some fat for body assimilation.

Power Food Program: Take two tablespoons of ordinary olive oil *before* you start any of your main meals. If you wish, add the oil to a raw vegetable salad which you eat at the start of the meal. The enzymes in the vegetables will then propel the oil throughout your digestive system, to lubricate and energize your gallbladder so it can function properly in food metabolism. You may also take the two tablespoons of olive oil in a glass of orange or grapefruit juice to make it easier to swallow. It's the gallbladder-pampering power food that helps keep it functioning smoothly and protects against gallstones.

THE "FREEDOM FROM GALLSTONES" POWER FOOD

Susan P. came from a family where most of the women had gallstones. Wanting to protect herself against this health risk, she asked her nutrition-minded physician about foods that would boost her resistance to gallstones. He suggested that she take at least four tablespoons of lecithin granules (from health store or pharmacy) daily. Susan P. follow this tasty advice. While others developed gallstones at age 40, Susan P. was well up in her early 60's and was free from this risk. She calls lecithin her "freedom from gallstones" power food.

How to Take Power Food: Sprinkle the lecithin granules over your fresh raw fruit or vegetable salads throughout the day. Or mix it in any fruit or vegetable juice, stir or blenderize and then drink slowly. Plan to take at least four tablespoons daily for protection.

Power Food Benefit: Lecithin, a soybean-derived power food, appears to improve the ability to digest and absorb fats because of its emulsifying abilities. It dissolves cholesterol deposits that might otherwise coagulate and crystallize to form stones. Its powerful benefit is that it can break fatty deposits into particles which can then pass readily through the tissues for body absorption. It is a power food that offers better gallbladder health and freedom from the risk of gallstones!

HERB TEA FOR GALLBLADDER HEALTH

Folklorists have always recommended drinking camomile tea as a means of stimulating the sluggish gallbladder so that accumulated sludge can be washed through the urinary tract and out of the body. To prepare, put one teaspoon of camomile (from health store or herbal pharmacy) into one cup of freshly boiled water. Add some lemon juice for Vitamin C action. Plan to drink as many as seven freshly prepared cups per day. Ingredients in the camomile herb become invigorated by the active Vitamin C from the lemon juice to promote a form of cleansing for the gallbladder.

Warm Olive Oil for Gallstone Expulsion. A folklore remedy for relief of gallstones is to lie down flat and in this position slowly sip half a cup of warm olive oil. The oil helps open the bile ducts to permit the passage of the gravels or stones for expulsion. Repeat several times during the day, if necessary, say folklore healers.

Basic Gallbladder Health Tips: Eliminate fried foods, rich pastries and gravies, pork, cream. Enjoy lean broiled or boiled meats, whole grains, fruits and vegetables and skim milk products. Drink lots and lots of water and fruit and vegetable juices daily. Avoid tension. Keep yourself physically and mentally active.

Gallbladder Cleansing Program. Use two ordinary power foods to help clean your gallbladder. Combine ½ cup of grapefruit (or lemon) juice with ½ cup of olive oil. Stir or blenderize, and drink down without delay. You would be wise to do this at night before going to bed. While you sleep, these two power foods start to work to help clean out your gallbladder of its old, thick and congested bile. In the morning, drink a glass of slightly warmed apple juice. Its malic acid content creates internal reverberations so that accumulated sludge and pebble-like encrustations can be washed out during your morning bowel movement. This simple program will do much to cleanse your gallbladder and help protect you against formation of gallstones.

Say goodbye to the fear of gallbladder distress with the use of these power foods.

See DIGESTIVE DISTURBANCES.

GOUT
Power foods that reduce swelling and restore health of joints

Gout is a metabolic ailment affecting the joints and kidneys. Body metabolism is out of kilter, resulting in more uric acid in the tissues than there ought to be. In an acute attack of gout, crystals of monosodium urate, a salt of uric acid, form in one or more joints, causing inflammation and severe pain. Gout causes periodic and sudden occurrence of very painful, swollen joints, particularly of the big toe.

Uric acid is manufactured in your body. It is produced from substances called purines which are found in many foods, but in especially large quantities in those which are the organs of animals, such as sweetbreads, brains, kidney and liver. Beer is another purine source.

Normally, uric acid is discharged from the body in the urine and intestinal tract and, in smaller quantities, through perspiration. But when body chemistry goes awry, uric acid becomes stored up in the blood and this precipitates a gout attack. Through the use of a corrective food program—and uric-acid-dissolving power foods—gout can be soothed and eased. The joints are restored to health and your entire body feels better.

THE SWEET POWER FOOD THAT HELPS WASH AWAY URIC ACID

Fresh red cherries are a deliciously sweet power food containing substances that can help dilute and weaken the pain-causing uric acid. Red cherries are able to prevent the crystallization of uric acid and make it easier for your metabolism to prepare it for excretion before it causes intense joint inflammation and pain. Eating a half pound or even a pound of pitted red cherries is recommended for gout healing.

Benefits: Red cherries have high concentrations of natural pigments, a balance of calcium and phosphorus together with high-powered potassium. These ingredients work in combination to wake up the sluggish metabolism to correct biological errors that have caused uric acid buildup.

Bonus Benefit: Power food cherries contain an enzyme which is able to form *uricase*, a metabolic ingredient which is needed to convert uric acid into the more soluble *allantoin* and thereby cause a healthy blood balance. It works to make allantoin, instead of uric acid, the end product of purine metabolism. Power food cherries help to convert uric acid into a more soluble substance for normal elimination.

Simple Program: Plan to eat a generous amount of freshly washed, pitted cherries regularly. They will give your biological metabolism the enzymes required for healthy uric acid balance. When your metabolism is corrected, there is less risk of swelling and greater opportunity for the restoration of the health of your joints.

Power Foods to Promote Gout Healing

- *Herb Tea.* Add one teaspoon of sarsaparilla leaves (health store or herbal pharmacy) to one cup freshly boiled water. Let steep for a few minutes. Flavor with a bit of honey and lemon juice. Plan to drink at least three freshly prepared cups each day. Ingredients in sarsaparilla tea are said to help boost sluggish metabolism, increase the flow of uric acid to eliminative channels, reduce painful swelling and improve joint health.
- *Mineral-Rich Chives.* This herbal garnish contains a high concentration of potassium, a mineral which pushes the uric acid out of the cells. This mineral works from *within* the cell and is able to promote cellular cleansing of the potentially harmful uric acid. Plan to eat chives as a garnish for your raw salad, in cottage cheese, yogurt, soups. They're refreshing and healthy.
- *Dandelion Tea.* This particular tea (use either dandelion root or leaves available from health stores and herbal pharmacies) contains high concentrations of substances that alert a sluggish circulation. This power food tea stimulates your red blood cells to flush out excess acid from the system. To prepare, just put one teaspoon of either the dandelion root or leaves in one cup freshly boiled water. Flavor with honey and lemon juice. Plan to drink at least three cups daily.

- *Celery-Carrot Juice.* Carotene is transformed by your digestive system into Vitamin A which combines with the potassium and phosphorus of the celery juice to help neutralize the corrosive burning effects of the stored-up uric acid. Your liver and kidneys respond beneficially, too. Plan to drink several glasses of this combination of power food juices daily to protect against gout and to create a more healthful uric acid balance.

Health Tips. Drink lots of liquids daily. Avoid purine-causing foods such as the organ meats described above: sweetbreads, brains, kidney, liver. Also avoid alcohol in all forms. Restrict your use of anchovies, sardines, meat extracts as in bouillons, gravies.

Bring down swelling and enjoy restoration of the health of your joints with the use of power foods and better health habits.

See Foot Problems, Leg and Foot Problems, Varicose Veins.

HAIR
Power foods that improve scalp health and promote hair growth

Hair growth depends largely upon a well-nourished blood supply reaching the roots in the scalp that are responsible for causing this growth. To discover how the use of power foods (internally and externally) can improve scalp health and promote hair growth, it helps to know some basic facts about hair and the way it grows.

Hair is actually a pigmented shaft that emerges from the hair follicle, a tubular opening in the outer layer of the scalp. Each follicle is a cluster of cells called the matrix. Hair grows from the follicular matrix. Your scalp and hair are nourished from the papilla, a microscopic nodule. This papilla is actually a part of the bulb-shaped skin membrane which surrounds the matrix. The papilla receives its hair-growing nutrients from your blood vessels and capillaries in and around your scalp.

A well-nourished scalp holds from 100,000 to 150,000 individual hairs. Each day, your scalp disposes of about 40 to 60 hairs which are replaced when your power-food-nourished papilla causes regrowth. It is when your scalp (and body) are malnourished that there is excessive hair fallout that is not adequately replaced and the thinning process takes place. With proper use of power foods and good scalp hygiene, you can nourish your body so that you will have a healthier growth of hair.

THE MINERAL THAT HELPS PROMOTE SCALP AND HAIR HEALTH

In his late 30's, Stuart Q. was embarrassed by his excessive hair loss. No matter what he tried, his hair started to thin out until he took to wearing a cap as often as possible. He discussed his hair loss with a dermotologist who was also a trichologist (hair specialist), and was told that he had a shortage of a little-known but powerful scalp-hair nourishing mineral—*sulfur*. The specialist boosted Stuart Q.'s sulfur intake through supplements and power foods. Within 19 days, his hair loss not only halted, but new growths appeared on his crown and at his temples. Within 40 days on this power food program, Stuart Q. had a healthy scalp and a healthy head of hair!

Power Food Hair Growing Program. Sulfur is a mineral that enters right into the scalp follicle, the papilla and the bulb portion to become part of the cell structure. Sulfur then releases important amino acids so that they can help reconstruct the follicles and nourish the cell walls and membranes to induce a better growth of hair. Sulfur is found in kale, watercress, Brussels sprouts, cabbage, cranberries, sorrel, turnips, cauliflower, raspberries, red cabbage, parsnips. Plan to eat these power foods daily, either raw (if possible) or cooked. You will be sending a high concentration of hair-growing sulfur to your scalp follicles.

Dandruff-Eliminating Power Food Scalp Wash. In a saucepan, place half a cup of apple cider vinegar, one cup of mint leaves and one cup of water. Boil slowly for five minutes. Remove from heat, strain and let cool. Then rub this power food mixture into your scalp. Using the soft parts of your fingers (don't scratch your scalp), massage gently and deeply for at least five minutes. Let remain overnight or longer. The high concentration of minerals in this scalp wash will help invigorate and nourish your sluggish papillae to induce a healthier scalp condition.

Protein Shampoo. Your scalp and its components as well as your hair itself consist largely of protein. By nourishing your scalp and hair with pure concentrated protein, you help stimulate better hair growth. To do so, try this power food *Protein Shampoo:* Beat two eggs (yolks and whites) together until fluffy. Now massage this fluff into your scalp with your fingertips. (Again, be careful not to scratch your scalp.) Massage for at least five minutes. Let this protein concentration seep into your scalp pores to nourish your papillae. Then rinse out with warmish water. (Not hot water or you may end up with a hair omelette!) Repeat nightly. Your scalp will become more protein nourished. Better scalp health leads to better hair growth.

Mayonnaise for Health-Plus Scalp-Hair Improvement. Ordinary mayonnaise is a powerhouse of vitamins, minerals and protein that become absorbed through your papillae to nourish the roots. To use this power food, all you have to do is first wash your hair. Now apply thick globs of this protein power food to your hair, and massage into your scalp. Let it remain for 30 to 45 minutes so ingredients can be absorbed. Then wash off with a little baby shampoo, warm and then cool water. Repeat regularly.

Eliminate Refined Carbohydrates. These include all refined sugar and sugar products. They tend to devour the important B-complex vitamins because of their too-rapid metabolic demands. Your skin (your scalp is skin, too!) needs the B-complex vitamins in order to keep itself healthy. Deprived of these vitamins, your skin may become dry, and when your scalp dries out it will not give you adequate hair growth. Switch to a bit of honey for sweetening; make sure all grains are fresh and natural. Read labels. Whole grain products are preferable since they are slowly metabolized and do not devour the B-complex vitamins which can then be used for skin-scalp-hair health!

Scalp-Hair Health Tips: Avoid damaging permanent waving, straightening or excessive bleaching. These procedures damage hair shaft and cause breakage of hair. Avoid the use of hot combs for styling. Tight hair styles cause tension that damages the follicles and leads to hair loss. As for rollers and clips, use foam-rubber instead of brush rollers. Use bobby pins with rubber tips. Avoid high heat which softens hair. Pat, instead of rub, your hair dry to avoid breakage. Use a soft, natural bristle brush (nylon bristles have rough ends) and brush gently. Wet hair should be groomed with a wide-toothed comb instead of a brush. Question use of certain scalp-injuring, hair-loosening drugs such as cortisone, blood thinners, amphetamines, antithyroid drugs, penicillin, mycin, sulfanomides. Avoid salt and salt-containing foods as this chemical appears to tighten hair follicles, causes tension, and chokes off hair growth.

The key to scalp health and hair growth is nourishment! This is found in power foods that improve your basic health and boost the growth of equally healthy scalp hair!

See SKIN.

HEADACHES
Power foods that relieve pain and soothe discomfort

More and more people seek treatments for headache than for any other common ailment. Headache is a complaint of the body against a condition of the mind. The pain is usually traced to some unpleasant or worrisome event or condition that causes anxiety. There is a feeling of constriction or "tightness" around the temples, in and around the eye sockets, the scalp, and just about the entire head. Severity varies so that pain and discomfort may be mild with some throbbing, or it may be so strong that the entire head is in agony, along with the rest of the body.

Headaches may occur regularly, intermittently, on and off—or rarely, if you are fortunate. But for most people, even an occasional headache can cause such discomfort that it can be disabling.

Basic Cause: Your brain interprets an ache from other parts of your body, but is itself unable to feel pain. The ache you feel involves the highly delicate nerve filaments (or nerve plexus) located inside the arteries that transmit blood to the brain. These nerve filaments or fibers are situated in the membranes comprising the inner and outer covering of the brain. They are very responsive to almost any stretch movement. When there is a bodily disorder, these delicate nerve filaments react and send transmission signals to your brain, which interprets the situation as a headache. To help correct this problem, improved living habits together with the use of specific soothing foods will be most beneficial.

POWER TONIC FOR SPEEDY HEADACHE RELIEF

To a glass of fruit or vegetable juice, add one tablespoon of brewer's yeast, one teaspoon of lecithin granules, one teaspoon of honey. Blenderize or stir vigorously until combined. Drink this and then rest in a chair in a cool, quiet room. Within one hour, your symptoms should subside and you will enjoy speedy headache relief.

Benefits: The brewer's yeast and lecithin granules are powerhouses of highly concentrated pyridoxine (Vitamin B_6) along with pantothenic acid and thiamin (Vitamin B_1). With the enzymes in the juice and the natural glucose in the honey, this combination almost immediately is transported via your bloodstream to soothe, calm and pamper your delicate nerve filaments. These delicate fibers will ease up on their spasms and reduce the transmission signals that are causing your pain. Swiftly, the signals stop and your brain is no longer attacked with these pain-causing vibrations. Within one hour, you should be able to say goodbye to the threat of a severe headache, with this easy-to-make and quick-to-act natural power tonic.

COOL "BURNING HEADACHES" WITH POWER GRAINS

Marie R. was plagued with recurring headaches. Long working hours and much pressure made her so tense that she would feel "burning headaches" that caused skin inflammation, nervous perspiring along with cold, clammy hands. Unable to take aspirins because of the threat of internal bleeding and digestive reaction, she asked her healer for any home remedy that would cool her "burning headaches" and ease distress. Her healer recommended a mixture of power grains, which he said would give her swift and lasting relief. Marie R. followed the program. Not only did her headache subside almost immediately, but she was soon rid of its recurrence and began to feel much better. She no longer had skin burning or perspiring. Circulation was improved so her hands felt nice and warm—thanks to the *Power Grains Headache Cooler.*

How to Prepare: To a glass of skim milk, add one tablespoon wheat germ, one tablespoon bran flakes, one tablespoon brewer's yeast. Blenderize or stir vigorously. Drink slowly. Rest in a cool, quiet room. The throbbing heat should ease up and cool off within 30 minutes. Other symptoms should begin to vanish in a few moments. Soon you'll feel relieved and in much better health.

Benefits of Power Grains Headache Cooler: The grains are highly concentrated sources of B-complex vitamins which combine with the soothing calcium and casein of the milk to restore normal flexibility to the dilated vessels involved in transporting blood through the body. These nutrients soothe the nerve cells. In a "hot headache," blood vessels in the membrane covering the brain are unable to dilate at uniform rates. Blood velocity passing through the smaller vessels is upset, causing painful dilation of the smaller vessels as they are forced to stretch to service the irregular arterial flow. This causes the "hot headache" reaction. But the *Power Grains Headache Cooler* offers a natural and speedy antidote by sending the high concentration of vitamins, mineral and casein (energizing protein) to correct vascular health and regulate even velocity of blood nourishment. By easing the dilation of the vessels, the pain is soothed and the "heat" is cooled off. This power food remedy works within 30 minutes to provide lasting relief. Whenever you feel the onset of a "hot headache" you should take this *Power Grains Headache Cooler*. It can be a welcome shield against pain.

SWEET POWER FOOD FOR HEAD PAIN RELIEF

Most headaches are traced to a drop in blood sugar. Correct this zigzag headache-causing reaction with a sweet power food that goes to work in a few minutes. Your pain vanishes, often as quickly as it began.

Cause: A drop in the sugar levels in your bloodstream prevents transfer of sufficient amounts of glucose into your brain. Starved for this nourishment, your brain reacts by sending forth distress signals. This is interpreted as pain. You feel it as a sudden headache.

Power Food Healer: Simple honey! This highly concentrated natural sweet is a powerhouse of glucose that is immediately absorbed by your bloodstream, transported to your brain for nourishment and relief of pain. Because honey is a pre-digested form of glucose, your metabolism is able to instantly propel it via your bloodstream to your starved brain. It works within a few minutes. In many headache situations, just take one or two tablespoons of honey. If you wish, brew a cup of herb tea and flavor with honey. You will feel instant relief as your glucose-nourished brain is contented and will no longer hurt you with pain signals.

Power Tonic for Speedy Relief. Take two tablespoons of apple cider vinegar, two teaspoons of honey and combine in a glass of plain water (or vegetable juice). Blenderize. Drink slowly.

Benefits: The potassium in the vinegar combines with the glucose of the honey to help regulate a soothing equilibrium between the intra- and extracellular fluids of your brain cells. This eases the pounding reaction of any balance disturbance. Within a half hour, this *Power Tonic* will soothe and erase headache distress via this cellular fluid balance.

Help your body nourish your vascular-brain system with power foods so that you will be able to enjoy pain relief and soothing comfort and so that headaches may be gone—forever!

See DIZZINESS, MUSCULAR ACHES, NECK PAINS.

HEARING PROBLEMS
Power foods that help correct hearing disorders

Hearing impairment results from varicose causative factors, either individually or in combination. Some of these audio-damaging factors include: cell-tissue degeneration because of viral infections, accidents which injure parts of the inner ear, arterial degeneration because of fatty buildup, nutritional disturbances that cause malfunctioning of the sensitive and specialized components situated within the inner ear which are responsible for accepting and dispatching sound to the brain's hearing center, and noise pollution.

In some situations, medications such as quinine and ordinary (but damaging) aspirins as well as antibiotics can cause a metabolic disorder that interferes with normal hearing and causes difficulties. Such medications may also lead to *tinnitus* or "ringing in the ears," which is your body's way of protesting the corrosive action of these chemicals.

First Step: Quiet Down. With noise will come hearing distress. Sonic pummeling is an assault upon the delicate mechanism of the hearing apparatus. Noise causes the tiny blood vessels involved in hearing to contract. Repeated noise pollution will keep them contracted so that they become stiff. This causes arterial injury; there is a subsequent increase in fatty materials in the bloodstream which cause clogging so that hearing becomes weaker and weaker. Not only will noise pollution dim your hearing, it can also cause erratic blood pressure, heart distress, neurological upset, among other things. It can become a chain reaction. Therefore, to keep your membranes flexible and your hearing (and body) in youthful health, quiet down. Shield yourself from the ravages of noise pollution. This is the first step in helping to prevent and correct hearing disorders.

POWER ELIXIR TO STRENGTHEN HEARING

Three nutrients, in a combined elixir, are able to help strengthen the arteries of the ear canal, those in the tympanic membrane and along the chain of ossicles to the inner ear and nerve. These segments of your ear are invigorated and rejuvenated when nourished with three specific nutrients. You can combine them in a glass of fruit and vegetable juice. Here's how:

In a favorite beverage, combine one tablespoon brewer's yeast, one tablespoon desiccated liver (from health store or pharmacy), one tablespoon of Vitamin C powder. (If not available in powder form, crush several tablets and add to this elixir.) Stir or blenderize. Then drink slowly.

Benefit: This *Power Elixir* is a concentrated source of the energizing B-complex vitamins—but more importantly, of *glutamic acid* (in the yeast and liver), which is a protein constituent that is eagerly needed for nourishment of the membranes and ossicles and related ear components as described above. These nutrients are energized and empowered by the Vitamin C to be transported speedily to the ear region to help repair damage and strengthen weakness. More important, the glutamic acid is used in combination with the two other nutrients to strengthen the tiny blood vessels that might otherwise become contracted and too stiff. The *Power Elixir* with the B-complex, glutamic acid and Vitamin C combo can help strengthen distorted arterial-vascular distress and promote better correction of hearing disorders. *Suggestion:* Drink one or two glasses of this *Power Elixir* daily to help your hearing and your body, too.

POWER OIL FOR IMPROVED HEARING

Gradual hearing loss made Michael U. extremely nervous. He felt much older than his middle 50's, especially when he had to cup his ear to listen to ordinary conversation. Such sounds as *k, g, p, t,* could hardly be heard—or not heard at all. Michael U. discussed his problems with his nutrition-minded otolaryngologist (specialist in hearing disorders) who observed that there could be a dietary cause. Michael U. was eating too many hard fats. He needed to wash out accumulated cholesterol deposits which were blocking his hearing. The otolaryngologist suggested a low animal fat program and a specific power oil that would help lubricate his hearing components and boost hearing. Michael U. followed this simple advice and took the power oil daily. Within 12 days, his hearing improved. Now he no longer had to strain his ears. The formerly indistinct letters such as *k, g, p, t,* came to him clearly. With the help of this power oil, his hearing was restored to that of a young person.

Power Oil: Wheat germ oil, taken as part of a salad dressing, or added to any vegetable juice and blenderized, offered a powerful artery-washing reaction that improved hearing. Wheat germ oil is a high concentration of Vitamin E which is the secret for better hearing. Take wheat germ oil (four to six tablespoons) daily!

Benefit: The Vitamin E and polyunsaturates in this power oil help to protect against the deterioration of fats, along the tympanic membrane and ossicular chain, which may cause hearing loss. This power oil also prevents excessive oxidation of cellular lipids and fatty peroxidation (interaction of oxygen and fat) which congest and degenerate delicate hearing nerves. In addition to using the *Power Oil* daily, go on a low animal fat program to help cleanse your arterial network of accumulated sludge. This improves your body health and will also help improve and correct your hearing powers.

Be good to your ears and you will be able to hear with youthful power and enjoyment.

See Ears.

HEART
Power foods that add years to your heart

When you use power foods to strengthen your heart, you reward the rest of your body with improved health and hope for a much longer life span. This master organ has the responsibility for doing more than just keeping you alive. It has the power to keep you youthfully alert in body and mind. Nourish your heart well, and it will give you better appearance, health and many more years of joyful living.

Heart Function: A well-nourished heart contracts and dilates about 72 times a minute, adding up to 100,000 times a day or nearly 40 million times a year. Your heart metabolizes up to half of your food into fuel to keep the rest of your body in youthful condition. It pumps blood from your veins into your arteries. It promotes the flow of oxygen to nourish your entire body from head to toe, regulates your temperature, becomes involved in emotional reactions. More than 4000 gallons of blood are pumped through your heart daily, to be used as a "river" transporting life and youth-building nutrients to every part of your body. Your blood pressure is also influenced by the health of your heart. As your "master pump," your heart needs power foods to help keep it functioning smoothly. To add years to your heart, here is a set of lifesaving and life-extending suggestions.

POWER FOOD PROGRAM FOR REJUVENATING YOUR HEART

The *basic* program is to protect your heart against ailment with a low saturated (hard) fat and low cholesterol food plan. Foods that should be limited include eggs, meats, butter and cream. These fatty foods tend to raise the level of cholesterol in the blood, contributing to the development of atherosclerosis. This condition is a type of hardening of the arteries in which deposits form inside the arteries and interfere with the free flow of blood *from, to* and *within* your heart. Denied ample blood-carrying nourishment, your heart becomes "choked," and this may give rise to heart distress. To avoid this life-shortening risk, follow this power food heart-rejuvenating program:

1. Eat no more than three egg yolks a week, including eggs used in cooking.
2. Limit your use of shellfish and organ meats.
3. Daily, eat 6 to 8 ounces of lean meat, fish or poultry, as desired. These are lower in saturated fat.
4. Choose lean cuts of meat. Trim visible fat. Discard the fat that cooks out of meat.
5. Avoid deep fat frying. Use cooking methods that help to remove fat—baking, boiling, broiling, roasting, stewing.
6. Eliminate your use of fatty "luncheon" and "variety" meats such as sausages and salami.
7. Instead of butter and other cooking fats that are solid (hydrogenated), use liquid vegetable oils and margarines that

are rich in artery-cleansing and heart-invigorating polyunsaturated fats.

8. Instead of dairy products made from whole milk and cream, used skimmed or low fat milk and cheese.

This 8-step *Heart Rejuvenating Program* is your foundation for boosting the health and vigor of your heart and entire body, too.

THE POWER VITAMIN THAT GIVES YOUR HEART NINE LIVES

With the use of a power vitamin, your heart is given a new lease for many more years of healthy life; in effect, this power vitamin can give your heart "nine lives" because it can counteract the effects of potential illness and offer you a protective shield against cardiac distress. The power vitamin is *Vitamin E.*

This power vitamin is able to:

1. *Revitalize Your Bloodstream.* Acts as a natural antithrombin (dissolves blood clots) in your bloodstream so that your heart is able to be nourished according to its needs to keep you youthfully healthy.
2. *Provide Energizing Oxygen.* A natural anti-oxidant in your body, it decreases the oxygen requirement of muscle by as much as 43 per cent. It creates a pathway for blood to get through the coronary artery. It helps prevent the occurrence of anoxia (lack of oxygen) which is the trigger that sets off anginal (heart) pain.
3. *Melt Internal Scar Tissue.* Helps create a metabolic reaction that both prevents and melts away unhealthy heart scar tissue. This strengthens and invigorates the heart so it can give you the desired "nine lives" benefit.
4. *Dilate Blood Vessels.* The power of Vitamin E is such that it is able to help open up new pathways in any circulation blockage, and dilate the blood vessels so that your heart is able to receive nourishing blood. It is able to bypass blocks produced by clots and hardened arteries which threaten

heart health. Vitamin E overcomes these barriers and transmits nutrient-carrying blood and oxygen right to the heart to give it many added years of youthful life.

How to Feed Power Vitamin to Your Heart. Use Vitamin E supplements, available at health stores and pharmacies. Plan to use these highly concentrated power food sources of Vitamin E: avocado oil, almond oil, corn oil, peanut oil, safflower seed oil, sesame seed oil, soybean oil, sunflower seed oil, wheat germ oil, linseed oil. Whole grain breads and cereals are high in this power vitamin for your heart. Wheat germ and bran are other extra-rich sources of essential Vitamin E. Use these foods daily. They help cleanse and correct disorders in your arterio-cardiac system to give "nine lives" to your heartline.

POWER FRUITS THAT ENERGIZE YOUR HEART

Citrus fruits (oranges, grapefruits, tangerines) are concentrated sources of Vitamin C, making them power fruits that are able to energize your heart.

Secret of Heart Energizing. When you eat citrus fruits, you release this power Vitamin C which is used speedily to form connective tissue and cells so that blood can go to and from (and within) your heart. Vitamin C is also used to heal fibrous scar formation, an integral part of heart health.

Special Benefit: The power fruits offer Vitamin C which encourages the synthesis in the arterial lining of substances known as *mucopolysaccharides*—a dynamic heart energizer as well as healer of any impending or pending disorders. This power Vitamin C also helps protect against arterial thrombosis, shielding your heart from injury.

Easy Way to Use Power Fruit: As often as possible, eat an assortment of seasonally available citrus fruits. Plan to eat a fresh grapefruit for breakfast, as well as a dessert . . . and even as an in-between snack. Oranges and tangerines are juicy good when eaten peeled (be sure to use the white string-like membrane which is a dynamic source of bioflavonoids, a Vitamin C derivative which is super-powerful in nourishing, cleansing, and most important, energizing your heart). *Suggestion:* Drink citrus fruit juices, singly or in combination, daily. You'll be supercharging your heart (and body) with vitality-producing Vitamin C.

THE GOLDEN POWER FRUIT FOR HEART REJUVENATION

The golden *banana* is a power fruit that contains a little-known but dynamically powerful substance that offers protection-plus for your heart. The substance is *potassium*, a mineral that is needed to strengthen your heart, boost neuromuscular function, improve its reflexes, invigorate its muscles and promote cellular growth and regeneration. Potassium enables your heart to pump blood with youthful force. It also enhances the myocardial tone, protects against permeability of cellular membranes which might otherwise cause edema (fluid saturation) and possible damage. The golden *banana* is a highly concentrated source of potassium, the heart-rejuvenating mineral.

Suggestion: Eat several bananas daily; either peeled out of the hand, or as part of a fruit or vegetable salad. Combine with citrus fruits for double-barrelled heart-saving benefits.

Add years to your heart with the aforedescribed power food program and the important individual power foods.

See ARTERIOSCLEROSIS

HEMORRHOIDS
Power foods that reduce swelling and provide cooling comfort

Hemorrhoids are varicose veins of the anal region. These are delicate veins which are affected by any intra-abdominal pressure including overweight and pregnancy but most frequently by straining at the stools and spending too much time at this body function. This unrelieved and repeated strain causes an enlargement and breakage of the blood vessels or the formation of blood clots as well as infectious scarring of the covering tissues.

If unrelieved, the hemorrhoids may continue to bleed and this may cause anemia. There is also the unpleasantness of painful irritation during passage of the stools. This may lead to the use of laxatives which can further aggravate the situation since they cause bowel irregularity and digestive-intestinal upset.

With the use of power foods, the condition of hemorrhoids should be eased so that swelling and inflammation subside. In many situations, corrective living programs with the use of power foods will help clear up the hemorrhoid condition.

THE 25¢ POWER FOOD THAT REDUCES HEMORRHOID DISCOMFORT

Troubled with constipation, Frank DeY. developed hemorrhoids which itched, irritated, and burned so much that it made life downright miserable for him. Frank DeY. had tried chemical preparations but they irritated his inflamed tissues and worsened the symptoms. He sought help from a urologist (physician specializing in elimination ailments) who suggested correcting the *cause* of the hemorrhoids—namely, constipation. With less stool straining, there would be a reduction and eventually an ending of the hemorrhoid problem. The urologist suggested using a simple, inexpensive power food that would help restore regularity in a matter of days. This power food was *ordinary bran!* Frank DeY. followed the doctor's advice. He took at least six to eight tablespoons daily, either in a cereal, mixed as part of a salad, or in baked goods. Within four days, he had conquered his constipation problem. Three days later, the hemorrhoid discomfort was reduced, along with the swelling. Now he felt comfortable again. Frank DeY. takes at least two to four tablespoons of this power food daily and is able to prevent a return of the constipation-causing hemorrhoids. This power food cost him 25¢ per week—for a lifetime of freedom from hemorrhoids.

What Is Bran? Bran is the coat of the seed of the cereal grain usually separated from the flour or meal by sifting or bolting. It contains hemicelluloses, pectic substances, mucilages and other compounds as well as lignin and cellulose. This makes it a bulk- or roughage- forming power food.

What Are Bran's Healing Benefits? As a cereal product, it is able to increase the water content of the wastes, producing bulkier but soft, well-formed stools. This leads to a balanced transit time in the gastrointestinal tract which is intermediate between being too rapid (causing diarrhea) or too slow (causing constipation). This increased volume and stool softening helps reduce strain which is a major factor in correcting and eliminating hemorrhoids.

How Can Bran Be Used? As part of any whole grain cereal; in soups, stews, casseroles, baking dishes; in salads both raw and cooked. Plain to use at least six tablespoons daily of this power food (available in all supermarkets, health stores) to help create regularity to guard against hemorrhoidal discomfort.

POWER FOODS FOR OVERNIGHT RELIEF OF SWELLING-BURNING DISCOMFORT

Try these two power food programs which should help relieve the swelling and/or burning of hemorrhoids:

1. Insert a peeled garlic clove into your rectum. Let it remain overnight. Soothing oils in the garlic penetrate the hemorrhoidal tissues to help relieve the swelling and cool the burning. Next morning, remove and discard the clove. You should feel much better. Repeat nightly until the problem appears to be totally resolved.
2. Insert a clove-sized whittled raw potato into your rectum. Let remain overnight. Minerals in the potato appear to reduce swelling and extinguish the agonizing, burning sensation. Next morning, remove and discard the potato. As in the preceding power food program, repeat nightly until the hemorrhoids have subsided.

Vitamin Soothers. Restore cellular strength with the application of Vitamin A and D ointments (from pharmacies and health stores). Let remain overnight. You may also try a Vitamin E suppository which helps to regenerate the irritated, burned tissues and promote healing relief. These are power vitamins that offer speedy relief and hope for freedom from hemorrhoids in a short time.

Basic Health Tips: Avoid unrelieved standing or sitting. Vary your position and posture. Shed overweight. Apply comfortably warm compresses. Bathe in warm water. Correct constipation. CAUTION: When you lift a heavy object (or cough heavily) you instinctively tighten your abdominal muscles and this squeezes your hemorrhoidal veins. Try this method: when you lift, breathe freely. This reduces abdominal pressure on the veins. Keep on breathing in and out. Do the same when at stool so you will not strain. Do *not* hold your breath when lifting or at stool or under any other circumstances. All these tips help to ease and even eliminate hemorrhoidal problems.

Power Food for Speedy Relief. Soak a piece of cotton with papaya juice and place against your rectum. This helps stop the bleeding of hemorrhoids in a short while. Let remain overnight to help bring down swelling and give you cooling comfort. *It works while you sleep!* Next morning, you should feel free of hemorrhoidal discomfort.

Follow basic programs to relieve constipation, rebuild your rectal area, and enjoy freedom from swollen, inflamed hemorrhoids!

See Colitis, Constipation, Diverticulosis.

INSOMNIA
Power foods that create natural sleep

Can't sleep? Worrying about insomnia is often more injurious than going without sleep! But you do need a good night's sleep. It helps rest all your organs, and restores better health to your processes of circulation, metabolism, digestion, muscular and respiratory systems. You will glow with more youthful health when you enjoy a good night of sleep. Your body organs will become regenerated so that you will be given many more years of youthful life. You will also have more resistance to many ailments when you invigorate and strengthen your body with regular refreshing and rejuvenating sleep.

What Is Insomnia? A condition in which you have a prolonged inability to enjoy sufficient sleep. An *occasional* bout with insomnia is no cause for alarm. But if you find that you cannot sleep at least three nights out of six, then you need to correct the situation with the use of everyday power foods

THE POWER BEVERAGE THAT HELPS YOU SLEEP IN 30 MINUTES

Whenever Judith V. cannot sleep, all she does is use a very simple, everyday power beverage. After drinking just one glass of this beverage, slightly warmed, she returns to bed and is fast asleep in 30 minutes or less. She awakens the next morning feeling refreshed and rejuvenated, thanks to this power beverage you probably have in your home right now.

This sleep-inducing power beverage is *milk!*

What This Power Beverage Will Do to Help You Sleep. Drinking a glass of plain warm milk will cause a large concentration of an amino acid known as *tryptophan*. This substance appears to help reduce the impulses from the recticular formation of your midbrain and thereby calm down your cerebral cortex, where most of the conscious activity of your brain takes place. (The reticular formation acts as a switching station between the highest levels of the brain and the rest of your nervous system. It seems to have the power of deciding when you are to be awake or asleep.)

Therefore, to induce natural sleep without chemical tranquilizers, drink milk in order to release *tryptophan* to help switch the reticular formation to sleep. Nervous impulses continue to circulate in the cortex and the rest of your brain, but *tryptophan* shields them from incoming impulses from the sense organs. It is this natural process that can make you naturally and healthfully sleepy within 30 minutes.

Suggestion: Just drink a slightly warmed glass of milk (use skim if you're fat-calorie watching) about an hour before bedtime. Its tryptophan is released speedily. You'll soon be enjoying healthful sleep. You'll feel great in the morning, too, because of the restful qualities of milk, a super-power beverage food.

HERBAL AND OTHER POWER FOODS TO HELP YOU SLEEP BETTER

Camomile Tea. This herbal tea creates a healthful and natural sedative effect upon the brain and induces a desire for sleep. Prepare a cup or two of camomile tea (flavored with lemon juice and honey) about an hour before bedtime. Ingredients in the herb will help you feel sleepy in a jiffy.

Violet Leaves Tea. This is flavorful herbal tea that you should inhale while sipping. Its fragrance seems to dull the senses and make you healthfully drowsy.

Use Calcium Foods. This mineral acts as a natural tranquilizer upon the nervous system, calming you down so you should be able to sleep better. It is found in dairy products, green leafy vegetables, and is very highly concentrated in *sesame seeds.* A handful of these seeds eaten an hour or two before bedtime, together with skim milk, gives you double-action power food benefits to help you sleep better.

Power Food Snack to Help You Sleep Better: Add one teaspoon of sesame seeds to a cup of plain yogurt. Stir and eat slowly.

Benefit: The calcium of the sesame seeds joins the *tryptophan* of the yogurt. In this combo, the nutrients enter your bloodstream and go to your brain where they become converted into *serotonin*, a substance that creates a balm-like effect to induce natural and refreshly healthy sleep.

Less Salt = More Sleep. Eliminate salt because it stimulates your system and leads to insomnia. Cells become electrified and "alarmed" when subjected to irritating salt. Switch to sea salt, a seaweed powder, or kelp or dulse as a substitute. These all contain minerals that help you sleep better.

With the use of these everyday power foods, you will help your body create natural sleep, an important function to help you enjoy better health and longer life.

See Muscular Aches, Neck Pains, Nervousness.

IRON (INSUFFICIENT)
Power foods that boost your iron supply

"Tired blood" is a common label for anemia, a condition that is brought on by an insufficient amount of iron available to the body. Without adequate iron, just about every part of your body struggles for oxygen. This may create such reactions as increasing fatigue, acid indigestion (heartburn), vertigo or dizziness, brittle fingernails, thinning hair, irritability, forms of itching, headaches, poor appetite, to name just a few. Iron is an important "power mineral" that is needed to help you enjoy better health and longer life.

Iron: Benefits of Power Mineral. This essential trace element is a vital constituent of every cell of your body. It is especially important to the oxygen-carrying cells of your muscles and blood. This power mineral is needed to help create hemoglobin, the oxygen transport pigment of your red blood cells. Myoglobin, the hemoglobin of muscle cells, cannot be formed without this power mineral. Neither can many valuable enzymes.

Problems of Shortage of Power Mineral. If your iron stores are depleted and your food program does not provide enough iron to meet your body's needs, then the amount of hemoglobin produced will drop. This causes the red blood cells to shrink and become pale. This is known as iron-deficiency anemia. If your body is progressively deficient in this power mineral, reactions include shortness of breath, weakness, pallor. The importance of iron is increased during the years of growth, pregnancy, nursing and menstruation. But adult women and men in the late middle years also show a need for increased iron because of a slow-up in the rate of metabolism. Therefore, you really never do outgrow your need for iron!

OFFICIAL POWER FOOD RECOMMENDATIONS FOR IRON BOOSTING

Physicians with the New York City Bureau of Nutrition have outlined a set of important power foods that will boost iron intake.[1] These specialists say, "Iron is an important mineral needed to make healthy blood. It combines with protein in the foods we eat to form hemoglobin, a substance in the blood which carries oxygen to all our tissues. *Iron is most efficiently used as a power mineral by the body when protein and high Vitamin C foods are eaten at the same time!*"

HIGH IRON FOODS

Liver,[2] kidney,[2] heart,[2] lean beef, nuts, high-iron cereals (check labels), prune juice, legumes (dry beans and dry peas, peanuts).

GOOD IRON FOODS

Eggs,[3] lean meats, poultry, tuna fish, sardines, whole grain bread and cereals, brown rice, sun-dried fruits, blueberries, dark green leafy vegetables (spinach, broccoli, escarole, collards, turnip tops, kale), green peas, green lima beans, tomato and juice, sweet potato, molasses.

IRON + PROTEIN + VITAMIN C = RICH BLOOD SUPPLY

When eating an iron food (listed above) combine it with a protein and a Vitamin C food from this list of official recommen-

[1]"Everybody Needs Iron," New York City Bureau of Nutrition, June, 1977.
[2]These foods are high in cholesterol so limit servings and portion sizes.
[3]Egg yolk is high in cholesterol so limit to three or four per week for adults.

dations to help boost the production of healthy red cells to give you a rich (and youthful) blood supply.

Protein Foods: Fish, poultry, lean meats, milk products (not butter, cream or cream cheese), organ meats such as liver, kidney, heart. (These organ meats are high in cholesterol so eat small servings.) Also include dried beans, peas, peanuts, peanut butter, nuts. NOTE: These are more effective in iron-building if you combine with another protein. Examples: kidney beans with meat, lima bean and cheese casserole. Also try kidney beans and rice, peanut butter and bread for good iron-building combinations.

Vitamin C Foods: Orange, grapefruit, tomato and juice, cantaloupe, strawberries, papaya, mango, guava, raw cabbage, green pepper, broccoli, cauliflower, Brussels sprouts, potato, collard greens, turnip greens, kale.

Effective Iron-Building Formula: Each day, select one or more items from your iron food list, your protein food list and your Vitamin C food list. Combine them, either raw or cooked, and eat in this mixture. It helps your body utilize as much iron as possible. The protein and Vitamin C foods contain natural magnets that help your body absorb and utilize the iron.

IRON-BOOSTING POWER TONIC

To a glass of citrus juice, add two tablespoons of desiccated liver powder (from health store or pharmacy), two tablespoons of brewer's yeast powder. Stir or blenderize. Drink slowly. You now have a powerhouse of an iron-boosting combination of iron, protein and Vitamin C in a unique combination. Within a few minutes, your metabolism takes this three-way combination, absorbs the iron into your blood through the upper part of your small intestine, stimulates production of red blood cells to help enrich your "rivers of life." Within 60 minutes, you'll feel comforting warmth surging through your body. Your skin will feel warm; you'll glow with youthful health; you'll now feel more invigorated as your entire body becomes more stimulated, awake and alive again! All this because you have given important iron to your body.

Eat Iron-Boosting Power Foods Daily. Plan to eat a combination of the important iron-boosting power foods daily: select from the preceding iron, protein and Vitamin C foods and enjoy them in *combination* at one meal to help enrich your bloodstream almost immediately.

Wake up your "tired blood" and enjoy better health with the use of these quick-acting power foods.

See BLOOD ENRICHMENT, CIRCULATION, WEAKNESS

ITCHING
Power foods that relieve nagging distress

Called *pruritis*, a skin itch is annoying because it is almost impossible to resist the urge to scratch. In so doing, you cause skin breakage. This worsens the condition. *Pruritis*, or itching without any visible lesions on the skin, is often traced to an internal distress that needs to be corrected to obtain relief.

Warning Signal: Itching is often a warning signal that there may be an underlying condition such as diabetes, anemia, gout, fungal skin infection. There may also be a reaction to certain foods and medications. Correct these causes and the itching symptoms should subside.

For generalized itching that may be traced to a skin rash, power foods (taken internally and externally) are able to help correct the neuro-dermatological disorder to give you relief from this nagging distress.

THE POWER OIL THAT ERASES STUBBORN ITCHING

Troubled with an annoying rectal itch, Herbert MacD. tried chemical preparations. They made his skin so irritated and inflamed, that they worsened his problem. He discussed it with his pharmacist, who recommended that he use an everyday "power oil" that should give him swift relief in a little while. That "power oil" was *wheat germ oil*. Herbert MacD. followed a simple program with wheat germ oil. Within two days, the itch was completely gone and he felt wonderful.

Simple, Effective Program. Follow the same program as outlined in this easy but effective two-step method:

1. Four Tablespoons Daily. Use four tablespoons of wheat germ oil (from health store or pharmacy) each day. Put on your raw vegetable salad. Stir in a glass of vegetable juice and drink slowly.

Benefit: The wheat germ oil is a power concentrate of important Vitamin E which has the power to help destroy harmful bacteria that may be responsible for your itch. Furthermore, it also helps establish a "beneficial bacteria" balance in your body so that the itch-causing fungi will be overcome and destroyed. This is the key to internal cleansing of the itch-causing elements.

2. Apply Wheat Germ Oil as an Ointment. Using mild soap and lukewarm water, wash the affected area. Rinse off, then dry with a soft towel. Now apply a coating of wheat germ oil as an ointment to the itching area. If possible, let remain overnight.

Benefit: The polyunsaturated fatty acids in the oil act as a "sealant" to your pores. They actually "choke" the harmful fungi and destroy them. The fatty acids also act as a soothing emollient to help ease the reddened, inflamed nerve endings that are causing the itch. Within a little while, the wheat germ oil will help soothe and calm the affected area so that you will soon feel immeasurably relieved.

Suggestion: Just follow this easy two-step "power oil" program for a few days and you'll discover relief and freedom from distressful itching.

POWER HEALERS FOR ITCHING

Prepare any of these power healers for easy use and speedy relief for itching anywhere on your body.

Power Ointment. Make a paste of baking soda and water. Apply to the freshly washed and dried itching area. Let remain overnight. Wash off and then re-apply. Itching should subside and vanish in a day or two.

Grain Poultice. Mix enough oatmeal and water to make a paste. Apply to the freshly washed and dried itching area. Let remain overnight. Wash off and then re-apply. The B-complex vitamins in the oatmeal soothe the nerve endings and thereby induce a feeling of soothing comfort within a short while. Itching should be healed in a day or two.

Power Juices. Just apply fresh lemon or lime juice or ordinary witch hazel for an occasional itch. The burning sensation becomes cooled in a matter of minutes.

Water + Salt = Itch Relief in Ten Minutes. Apply some cool water to the exact itching area. Let it dry. Now rub in a few grains of salt. Rub and rub until you feel the itching going away. For any stubborn itch, this water and salt rub combination will help provide soothing relief within ten minutes.

POWER FOODS TO PROTECT AGAINST ITCHING

Boost your intake of power foods that are high in the important B-complex vitamins. These nutrients will help soothe the irritated nerve fibers so that there is less skin sensitivity and reaction.

Power Food Sources of B-Complex Vitamins. Whole grain breads and cereals, wheat germ, bran, lentils, kidney beans, spinach, collards, dandelion greens, cabbage, cauliflower, cheddar cheese, salmon. Plan to eat some of these daily to fortify yourself against recurring itching.

Power Fruit Juice for Swift Relief. If body perspiration causes irritating itching, drink several glasses of any *citrus fruit* every day. You may also eat the citrus fruit itself, as a snack or as part of a salad as well as a dessert.

Healing Benefit: Citrus fruits and their juices contain high concentrations of Vitamin C. This power vitamin acts as a hydrogen ion carrier for those enzyme systems involved in the perspiration glands.

During excessive sweating, a shortage of Vitamin C appears to develop; the enzyme cannot function properly. This leads to that annoying itch. Supplement this Vitamin C-enzyme deficiency by drinking citrus fruit juices often. Build up more than just healing powers—build up immunity reactions to that annoying and distressful itch!

You will look and feel much better without that constant itch. Use these power food programs to help improve resistance and promote swifter healing for nagging itching.

See SKIN.

JAUNDICE
Power foods that restore your bile balance and healthy skin color

Jaundice is a greenish-yellow or yellow tinging of the skin. This discoloration may also appear in the white and conjunctive tissues of the eyes. Jaundice manifests itself in the clay-color of the stools. This is not an ailment but a symptom. It occurs if the liver becomes sluggish and bile pigments accumulate within the bloodstream, giving the skin its yellowish color. Jaundice may be a symptom of an ailment that is destroying the red blood cells, an obstruction in the gallbladder, a fatty buildup in the liver itself, retaining the pigments that should be eliminated.

To help restore bile balance and a normal, healthy skin color, the use of power foods will stimulate the sluggish liver and at the same time cause a release of stored-up bile pigments in the bloodstream.

POWER JUICE TO PROMOTE BETTER BILE FLOW

Combine a half-cup of sauerkraut juice with a half-cup of tomato juice. Stir and then sip slowly. Plan to drink at least three glasses of this power juice daily. For more effective bile-distributing powers, go on a simple one- or two-day controlled fasting program.

During this time, limit nourishment solely to this power juice. Your digestive enzymes will now be able to work without interference of other nutrients. The enzymes will take up the high concentration of Vitamin C along with the fat-metabolizing B-complex vitamins in both the sauerkraut and tomato juices, and promote better distribution throughout your body. Just three glasses in one day will help break down and release stored-up bile concentrations in the bloodstream for body distribution. It may also help to create "overnight" bile balance and restoration of youthful skin color and body health.

Power Tonic for Freedom from Bile Blockage. Just two power foods are able to create an internal rejuvenation whereby bile that is blocked or in a backup stagnation in your bloodstream can be released from congestion and sped on through normal eliminative channels.

These two power foods are *brewer's yeast powder* and *lecithin*. Both are high concentrates of essential B-complex vitamins which stimulate the activity of the gallbladder and liver to promote better emptying, to break up the bile particles into a form that will create better distribution.

Power Tonic: In a glass of fresh orange or grapefruit juice, stir two tablespoons each of brewer's yeast powder and lecithin. If possible, blenderize for better assimilation. Drink three freshly prepared power tonics daily. Almost immediately, the vitalic B-complex vitamins will help to break down the congestion in your bloodstream, restoring a healthier flow of your bile so that you will not run the risk of jaundice.

Wheat Germ Oil for Better Bile Balance. This nut-like tasty oil, used as part of a salad dressing or combined with a tart fruit juice as a tonic, has the power to create better bile balance in your bloodstream, often within a few days.

Benefits: Wheat germ oil is a powerhouse of Vitamin E which helps break down the accumulated bile pigments and then distribute them more freely throughout your bloodstream. Vitamin E is the active principle in your bloodstream that propels the distributed bile to the normal eliminative channels. *Suggestion:* Add at least four tablespoons of Vitamin E-rich wheat germ oil to your daily raw salad. Combine with a little apple cider vinegar for better taste. Add this wheat germ oil to any desired tart juice. Four tablespoons to an eight-ounce glass daily will help boost internal energy and correct sluggishness that may cause this bile stagnation, the threat of jaundice.

Basic Health Tips: Increase intake of fresh fruits and vegetables along with their juices. They are powerhouses of needed enzymes, vitamins and minerals that will stimulate sluggish organs to facilitate a healthier bile balance. Enjoy whole grain breads and cereals as well as seeds and nuts because of their high B-complex values. This vitamin group is needed to help revitalize your bile-making and bile-distributing gallbladder and liver. Avoid alcohol and tobacco because these toxic habits tend to erode blood cells and may lead to "spillover" of accumulated bile.

With proper health care and the use of power tonics, you should be able to enjoy a better bile balance, a healthier skin color and a much more enjoyable and youthful life style!

See Digestive Disturbances, Gallbladder, Kidneys, Liver, Urinary Problems.

KIDNEYS
Power foods that rejuvenate your kidney's filtering powers

These dynamic organs, your kidneys, have the awesome responsibility of purifying over one ton of blood daily! Your kidneys also need to regulate your body's fluid balance and maintain the proper amount of water in your blood and elsewhere in your body at every single moment—whether you are awake or asleep.

Your kidneys produce hormones and enzymes which interact

with similar substances produced elsewhere in your body so that you are able to maintain a healthy blood pressure.

Furthermore, these two-bean shaped organs, each about the size of a clenched fist, situated near the lower ribs in your back on either side of your spine, need to maintain a delicate acid-alkaline balance. These organs are protected by a fatty layer and a glove of connective tissue that helps keep them in good position.

As your body's filtering organs, your kidneys need to anticipate the requirement to eliminate urea, phosphates, oxalates, wastes and ammonia, around the clock. They must also "know" how to retain exactly the right amount of vitamins and minerals. Any upset may cause general body upset and a risk of such ailments as nephritis, acute kidney infection and kidney stones, as well as uremia.

Headache, Nausea, Scanty Urine. These symptoms usually suggest that something has disturbed the health of your body's filtering organs. Your upset kidneys react by causing recurring headaches and nausea as well as appetite loss; urine is scanty and/or smoky. There may be a rise in blood pressure. In some situations, a disturbed kidney "complains" by giving you edema (swelling of the body). Your face or ankles become puffed up. You may even feel a mild ache in your kidney region. Your tongue may be discolored or "furred." To help calm down your "outraged" kidneys, use power foods to promote better distribution of liquids and improve the important filtering power.

THE POWER LIQUID THAT HELPS "STEAM CLEAN" YOUR KIDNEYS

Steam, in the form of heated water, has the power to cleanse and detoxify your clogged-up kidneys. This is a power liquid program that costs nothing and takes only 30 minutes a day, but may give you immediate relief and healing of your upset kidneys.

How to Take Steam-Cleaning Program: Turn on the boiling hot water in your bathtub. Let it fill up your tub while you remain seated on a stool in the closed bathroom. (Stay out of drafts. All doors and windows must be shut tight.) Just 30 minutes, as the sweat comes pouring out of your steam-opened pores, will create powerful cleansing of your kidneys and other organs, too. After this 30-minute program, towel-dry yourself and put on a warm robe. Lie down in a warm (draft-free) bedroom and rest for an hour. (Remember to drain the hot water from the tub.)

Benefits: This steam-cleaning program helps your kidneys flush out accumulated wastes from your bloodstream. In particular, the perspiration induced by the steam tends to increase release of backed up *urea nitrogen*. This waste product is usually passed off in urine but if your kidneys are sluggish, it remains in the bloodstream and this may cause internal toxemia. But the steam cleaning that uses an *absolutely free* power liquid—water—helps promote better release of this toxic substance and thereby keep your body clean and your kidneys in efficient filtering condition.

Suggestion: Just one 30-minute steam-clean program a night for three nights will help rejuvenate your kidney's filtering powers.

THE POWER FOOD THAT PROTECTS AGAINST KIDNEY STONE FORMATION

A power food mineral, *magnesium,* is able to rejuvenate your kidneys and create an internal reaction that helps protect against the threat of kidney stone formation.

Power of Magnesium. As a power mineral, magnesium is able to make your urine more solvent in regard to oxalates, the major substance that makes up kidney stones. Magnesium creates this greater solvency reaction so that your body fluids can hold the oxalate crystals with much less risk of aggregation or precipitation, or the clumping together of stone-forming particles. Magnesium alerts your kidneys to create more activity so that oxalates in the urine become filtered out and then broken down so that they can be released through normal eliminative channels. This process is made possible when your kidneys are adequately nourished with this power mineral.

Kidney-Feeding Magnesium Sources: Milk, nuts, whole grains, green vegetables, particularly as part of the chlorophyll molecule. Seafoods are also good sources of this kidney-feeding power mineral.

Power Food Supplement for Kidney Rejuvenation. Boost the filtering powers of your kidneys by taking *dolomite*, a naturally occurring mixture of magnesium together with calcium. Available at health stores and pharmacies, dolomite is a power food supplement that will rejuvenate and invigorate your kidneys to help create a urine solvency reaction that protects against stone formation. Plan to take 500 milligrams daily for good health and protection.

Power Foods from Folklore. To keep your kidneys sparkling clean, here are reported folklore power foods:

- *Parsley Tea:* Into a cup of freshly boiled water, place a punch of parsley. Let it cool. Remove parsley. Flavor with lemon juice and honey. Sip several freshly prepared cups of parsley tea as a healthful kidney-revitalizing power beverage.
- *Cranberry Juice:* The high concentration of Vitamin C together with enzymes in the cranberry appear energizing to the kidneys. Drink several glasses of cranberry juice daily for total health.
- *Asparagus:* The magnesium and Vitamin A content of this power food makes it cleansing and soothing to the kidneys. Steamed asparagus flavored with herbs and spices and a bit of oil will help improve kidney and body health. Tastes powerfully good, too.
- *Camomile Tea:* This herb tea is believed to help dissolve oxalic acid accumulations and dilute the concentrations that may cause formation of kidney stones. Drink several cups of this flavorful tea daily.

With the use of these helpful power foods, you should be able to "steam clean" and refresh, rejuvenate, and regenerate your kidneys, and enjoy a filter-clean bill of health from head to toe!

See Jaundice, Liver, Weakness.

LEG AND FOOT PROBLEMS
Power foods that improve flexibility and relieve congestion

A pain or cramp in the thigh or leg can be so upsetting that it forces you to suspend all normal activity. If such a pain progresses, it may seize hold of the entire leg, from the thigh right down to the toes themselves. This causes difficulties in sitting, standing and walking. Leg and foot problems tend to involve other body parts so that there is a feeling of generalized weakness and fatigue. This may lead to general body exhaustion and premature aging since functions become restricted or limited.

These pains need not occur only when you are in motion. They may be felt at night while you are trying to sleep. Even when you remain immobile, hoping to take pressure away from painful muscles, the spasms keep recurring so that you are not able to obtain adequate rest. This worsens your health condition and the symptoms seem more painful as time goes on. To help make you feel better all over, you need to improve the flexibility of your lower limbs and relieve pain-causing congestion. With the help of power foods, you should be able to revive "starved" leg and foot muscles, nourishing them to better strength and more youthful health.

THE POWER OIL THAT CALMS NOCTURNAL LEG CRAMPS

Wheat germ oil, a high-concentrated source of Vitamin E, is able to help calm down the health-destroying problem of nocturnal leg cramps. In this condition, there are painful spasms and aches in your calf and thigh muscles that cause intense pain during the night, when you should be getting needed sleep. With the use of Vitamin E-rich wheat germ oil, you should be able to help ease these spasms and do away with leg cramps.

How Power Oil Healed Stenographer's Nightly Distress. As an office stenographer, Evelyn LaD. divided her working time between sitting, standing, walking, doing various chores. Yet she was constantly plagued with knife-like pains shooting through her calf muscles and up to her thighs. Sitting offered little relief. At night, the leg cramps were so severe she would cry out as the pain knotted her muscles. Desperately, she asked a nutrition-minded physician for help since medications gave her many side effects. He suggested she take at least 500 units daily of Vitamin E, either in the form of a food supplement or wheat germ oil. The dosage could be easily calculated by following label directions. Evelyn LaD. began to take this amount daily. Within four days, her pains subsided, then vanished. Now she felt rejuvenated flexibility in her legs as she sat, stood, walked or ran. She could sleep the night through without these nocturnal leg cramps. The power oil had made her legs (and body) feel young again!

Healing Power of Vitamin E. This nutrient tends to invigorate leg muscles to increase circulation, free muscles and joints from obstructions and thereby boost the flow of blood-carrying oxygen to the injured, pained areas. This process appears to help restore more youthful flexibility to the limbs and the body, too. Whether in the form of Vitamin E (from health store or pharmacy) or wheat germ oil, this power oil is able to promote swift, effective healing of leg pains.

Power Tonic for "Young Forever" Legs and Feet. Help loosen up your "aging" leg muscles and pained feet with this easy-to-prepare but highly effective power tonic. In a glass of fruit juice, mix one tablespoon of non-fat dry milk powder, one tablespoon of apple cider vinegar, one teaspoon of lecithin. Blenderize or stir vigorously. Drink this *Power Tonic for "Young Forever" Legs and Feet* about two hours before bedtime. You will be able to enjoy a refreshing night of sleep without the "restless legs syndrome" problem. After two or three nights, this power tonic will have done away with the painful problems.

Benefits: The enzymes of the fruit juice combine with the calcium and protein of the milk, become energized by the vinegar and invigorated by the protein of lecithin. This combination boosts a unique *calcium assimilation* within your bone structure so that your leg muscles are calmed down, the cramps are soothed and there is improved flexibility. This power tonic works swiftly. Within a few hours, you feel soothed and relaxed. You'll be able to sleep better. Your legs will become rejuvenated by morning. You'll awaken to greet the day with energy, vitality, and, most important, ache-free legs.

Power Food Supplement. Health stores and pharmacies have *calcium lactate*, a unique power food supplement which is able to soothe the nerves and tissues of your limbs, almost within minutes. This power food supplement is absorbed into your bloodstream where it is then able to act as a balm of contentment for your frazzled pain-causing muscle cells. Take it with fruit or vegetable juice whenever you feel the beginning of pain. You'll obtain energetic relief almost at once.

There is no need to feel panic because of leg and foot problems. With the use of power foods, you can help correct the causes and enjoy better flexibility and congestion-free youth of your limbs and your entire body.

See Foot Problems, Muscular Aches, Stiffness, Varicose Veins.

LIVER
Power foods that invigorate liver-detoxifying functions

A well-functioning clean liver is essential for better health and longer life. After your skin, the liver is the second largest (about four pounds in weight) organ of your body. As a metabolically versatile organ, your liver performs more essential health- and life-producing functions than any other part of your body.

Liver: Key to Improved Youthful Health. A power food-invigorated liver is able to manufacture the blood-clotting agents, prothrombin and fibrinogen, without which we would bleed to death from the slightest wound. A healthy liver produces and stores glycogen, a source of glucose energy needed by both the brain and muscles. A healthy liver is needed to create bile, an important substance basic to the digestion of fats. The liver also helps in the metabolism of minerals, proteins and energy-producing carbohydrates. A valuable function of the liver is to detoxify noxious chemicals that find their way into the body. It also is needed for the storage of Vitamins A, B, D, E and K. This master organ of your body makes its own enzymes which work on amino acids and carbohydrates as soon as they arrive, rearranging them into new and usable proteins to help keep your entire body in youthful health. Its major health-building function is to filter out poisons and wastes and thereby protect the body from internal toxemia. If this filtering-detoxifying function is impaired, then the entire body loses health. Ailments range from malaise, weakness, muscle-mental weakness to hepatitis and cirrhosis of the liver. To protect against liver disorders, power foods will help improve its filtering processes.

Healthy Liver = Healthy Gallbladder. Situated in the upper abdomen, mostly on the right side just beneath the diaphragm or food gullet, the liver manufactures and releases bile for digestion; this bile is stored in the gallbladder. A healthy liver will release healthy bile to the gallbladder, which in turn is nourished by its neighboring organ. But if the liver malfunctions or otherwise releases toxin-laden bile to the gallbladder, then the adjacent organ becomes ill and there is the risk of declining health. To enjoy healthy body organs, improve the vigor and filtering power of the liver.

PROTEIN POWER FOODS FOR CLEAN LIVER

Andrew C.C. started to develop headaches and sore muscles. His appetite became poor. His skin took on a sallow look. At times, he had arthritic-like pains shooting through his fingers and arms. He walked with a stooped, prematurely aged gait. Taking his problems to his family endocrinologist, he told how he had been smoking, drinking a lot, and eating "fast" foods. Andrew C.C. was put on a protein power food program after he was told that his unhealthy living habits were weakening the filtering powers of his liver. Instead of cleansing out wastes, there was a backup and buildup of bile; this was causing his dark-colored urine and occasional diarrhea, together with his other reactions. The protein power food program, together with correction of improper and liver-abusing habits, soon put him back on the road to health. Andrew C.C.'s face glowed with health, his pains were gone, he walked erect, his urine was normal-colored and his diarrhea disappeared. He recovered within four days on this protein power food program. It cleaned and regenerated his abused liver and made him look and feel young again.

Protein Power Program: Boost daily intake of lean and fat-trimmed meats, skim dairy products, fish, seeds, beans, nuts. Each day, have a raw vegetable salad with a dressing to which you add high-protein wheat germ or lecithin or both. Give up smoking and drinking. Limit or restrict "processed foods" which may be "fast" but are low in important nutrients and high in liver-clogging refined carbohydrates.

Daily Liver-Regenerating Tonic: To a glass of vegetable or fruit juice, add two tablespoons of high-protein brewer's yeast, two tablespoons of wheat germ, one tablespoon of lecithin, one tablespoon of non-fat dry skim milk powder. Add a bit of honey. Blenderize. Drink up to three freshly prepared glasses of this *Liver-Regenerating Tonic* each day.

Benefit: The high protein of the yeast and lecithin and milk become invigorated by the energy-creating natural carbohydates and B-complex vitamins of the grains and create an internal flushing of the filtering components of the liver. At the same time, the liver will use the amino acids of this tonic to create self-regeneration of its cells and tissues so that this master filter quickly becomes rejuvenated. This is a power tonic that adds years of healthy life to the filtering powers of your liver.

THE POWER VITAMIN THAT SPEED-CLEANS THE LIVER

Choline, a lesser-known but extremely powerful B-complex vitamin, is able to speed-clean the liver by boosting the metabolism of ingested fats that must be dispersed through this organ. Choline energizes the liver to metabolize ingested fats into the form of phospholipids and burn them up in the form of usable fatty acids.

Caution: Without sufficient amounts of this power vitamin, the liver cells are not able to cleanse themselves of fatty acids which are brought to them by the bloodstream. Fat droplets may now settle within the liver cells to form sludge-like structures. This fatty infiltration reduces the liver's power to detoxify substances that enter the bloodstream, to metabolize proteins and carbohydrates or to balance electrolyte levels in the body's tissues. If choline is continuously deficient, then the clogged liver is unable to eliminate poisons. The entire body may become infected. To protect against this liver clogging, the power vitamin choline is vital for total body health.

Sources of Power Vitamin. Whole grain foods, egg yolks (high in cholesterol), some meats and fish. A highly concentrated source of choline is found in *lecithin.* This soybean food is able to deliver a dynamic amount of choline to your liver where it immediately cleanses and helps dissolve accumulated and infiltrated fatty sludge that may be lodged in your liver lobules. By dissolving these fatty droplets, lecithin is able to help cleanse your liver and reduce the age-causing problem of steatosis (fatty accumulations).

Liver-Cleansing Program: Use up to five or six tablespoons of lecithin granules daily (from health store or pharmacy). Add it to whole grain cereals, to soups, stews, baked goods, casseroles. Dissolve it in juices for a healthy liver-cleansing and choline-high tonic. Combine with brewer's yeast for an invigorating liver-cleansing reaction in a fruit or vegetable juice. Be choline-good to your liver through lecithin and your whole system will respond with total detoxification and a clean bill of health.

Keep your liver clean and you will enjoy better health inside and outside your entire body.

See Gallbladder, Jaundice, Kidneys.

LOW BLOOD SUGAR (HYPOGLYCEMIA)
Power foods that establish vital energy balance

For youthful energy, your body must have a balanced supply of glucose. This is a blood sugar which feeds your brain, regulates the hormone-producing functions of many of your glands, improves the function of your muscles and helps to correct so-called "aging" or chronic fatigue of body organs and muscles. A deficiency or reduction of this important substance will cause low blood sugar or hypoglycemia.

Hypoglycemia may also be a reaction of an ailing liver if that master organ is unable to produce sufficient amounts of glucose. Therefore, a healthy liver is important for maintaining healthy glucose levels.

Hypoglycemia may also be the result of a sluggishness of the glucoreceptors in the central area of the hypothalamus (an endocrine gland involved in the functions of the autonomic nervous system.)

Normally, the glucose blood level is maintained at a fairly constant level, between 60 to 100 milligrams per 100 milliliters of blood. If there is a drop in this level that is not relieved, then hypoglycemia results.

Weakness, Shaking, Irrational Behavior. A low blood sugar condition causes such reactions as severe weakness, dizziness, uncontrollable shaking, emotional instability, sweating, blurred vision, even blackout spells. Unrelieved hypoglycemia may cause convulsions and coma.

THE BASIC POWER FOOD PROGRAM FOR SPEEDY ENERGY BALANCE

Follow this simple but highly effective energy-boosting program to help restore a good glucose level in your bloodstream.

1. *Eliminate Refined Carbohydrates.* These include processed grains, cakes, pies, pastries, candies, sweets of all sorts. They offer you predigested carbohydrates which give you a quick energy boost but this is followed with a severe letdown when these sugars and starches are metabolized. You'll become victim of a seesaw or yo-yo tug of war, going from speedy energy to complete exhaustion. Eliminate these non-foods.
2. *Boost Intake of High-Protein Foods.* These include lean meats, fish, dairy products, beans, peas, nuts, seeds. Plan to eat an ample portion of these high-protein foods daily.

By following this program, you'll be able to stabilize your blood glucose levels within minutes and be rewarded with a speedy but long-lasting energy balance.

Energy-Boosting Snacks That Work in Minutes. Whenever Betty McK. feels weak, whether waiting on line or while driving, she reaches into her handbag and takes out an energy-boosting snack. Sun-dried fruit! This could be raisins, pitted dates, figs, prunes, grapes. These sun-dried fruits are a powerful concentration of *natural sucrose*, and eating a handful of them will give Betty McK. a terrific surge of youthful energy—within minutes. She has solved her recurring bouts of hypoglycemia with this power food energy snack program.

Power Protein for Better Blood Sugar Balance. High protein foods such as lean meats (try a chicken or turkey drumstick), cheese chunks, a hard-boiled egg, cup of cottage cheese, a handful of shelled seeds and nuts. Eating a half-cup of walnut meats will give you a high concentration of protein that is balanced with polyunsaturated fatty acids to create a *slow metabolism* so that your bloodstream is "fed" a steady supply of glucose to provide you with refreshing energy in a regulated balance. Just carry any of these high-protein foods with you and munch when you feel the need for an energy boost.

Eat a Good Breakfast. Power foods would include any of the above-mentioned protein items. These power foods do not overload your blood with sugar but send glucose first to the liver so it can dole out the glucose as it is needed. This prevents overloading in your bloodstream. You'll have day-long energy if you alert your sluggish blood sugar levels with these protein power foods in the morning. *Bonus Benefit:* Calories consumed in the morning are more easily and speedily converted into *energy* than are calories consumed before bedtime, which are converted into *extra pounds.*

Brewer's Yeast for Energy Boost. In a glass of vegetable juice, stir two tablespoons of brewer's yeast. Drink slowly. You'll feel a surge of vitality within moments.

Benefits: This power food is high in chromium, a trace mineral which helps establish vital energy balance. This power mineral helps raise the glucose levels to release a slow but steady energy-producing factor. Plan to drink three glasses daily of this "instant energy" elixir. The chromium is a power mineral that will give you a surge of long-lasting youthful vitality. It works within minutes.

Be young in mind and body with a balanced blood sugar level made possible with the help of everyday power foods.

See DIZZINESS, FAINTING, IRON, "SWEET TOOTH," WEAKNESS.

MENTAL ALERTNESS
Power foods that protect against senility and revitalize thinking

A vigorous mind made possible by the brain-activating principles found in power foods will do much to help you enjoy more than just a longer life span. It will also help you "think young" and "live young" in mind and in body.

Oxygen Starvation Is Cause of Senility. Deprived of sufficient oxygen, the brain tissues start to choke. This will cause mental confusion, disorientation and poor memory—the symptoms of the condition usually called senility.

The problem here is that the peripheral blood vessels (microscopic capillaries spread throughout the brain) start to become narrow or constricted. This lowers the supply of oxygen available to the brain cells and tissues and leads to what is known as senility.

To help correct this cause and to do more than just protect against senility by revitalizing your thinking capacities and boosting your mental alertness, power foods can help you roll back your mental years and give you the responsiveness of a healthy young person.

FROM "DOPE" TO "BRIGHT" IN NINE DAYS

Stephen E. R. started to have memory lapses. In his middle 60's he could not remember his telephone number and had to look it up in his wallet. He forgot the names of his children and confused one with the other. Quite often, he was found wandering around the streets of his home town, unable to know how to get back to his residence. The local missing person's bureau was always scouting around to find out where he had become lost. Stephen E. R. might have been put in an old people's home, even at his comparatively young age, because his family feared for his safety, except that a local geriatrician (specialist in ailments of older people) noted that he had a serious nutritional deficiency. He recommended the use of just *one* power vitamin in an easily available food, and with this vitamin Stephen E.R. was able to recover. Within nine days, the "dope" (as some unkind people called him) became "bright" and very much alert. A few days more and he was so energetic he decided to take a part-time job to keep active, even if he was retired. Stephen E.R. takes this power vitamin food daily. He calls it his "brain food."

THE POWER VITAMIN FOOD THAT REVITALIZES THINKING ABILITIES

Choline, a member of the B-complex vitamin family, found in high concentrations in lecithin, a soybean-derived food, is the key to the revitalization of thinking. It helped Stephen E. R. discover new life in nine days. It is the key to dynamic mind power.

Benefits: Choline, as found in lecithin, is able to penetrate the so-called blood-brain barrier, to pass directly into the brain cells. Here, this power vitamin stimulates these cells to release more acetylcholine (a substance that is involved in the transmission of nerve impulses) and to help improve thinking as well as revitalize memory.

Boost Mental Alertness with Choline

Include an ample amount of choline and you will enjoy more youthful brain power and improved memory, according to medical studies.[1]

Dr. Richard J. Wurtman of the Massachusetts Institute of Technology (MIT) says that choline from food passes into the blood from

[1] *Natural Health Bulletin*, Parker Publishing Company, West Nyack, New York 10994. October 8, 1978, Volume 8, No. 21. Available by subscription.

the digestive tract and then is taken up directly by the brain from the circulating blood.

Boosts Brain Function. "Its main function is to provide your brain with acetylcholine, to aid your brain in making an important chemical transmitter of nerve signals. On an hour-to-hour basis, the amount of nerve signal transmitter in the brain seems to depend upon how much choline-rich food an individual has recently eaten."

Works Swiftly. Says Dr. Wurtman, "The person who eats foods with a high choline content will, within a few hours, have an extra supply of the nerve signal transmitter, acetylcholine, in the brain. This means an *amplification* of the signals sent from one nerve cell to the next." This power vitamin is identified as the "active principle" involved in creating mental alertness and better brain-memory responses.

How to Use Power Vitamin. Lecithin granules, from health store or pharmacy, are high concentrations of choline, the brain-boosting power vitamin. Plan to take from four to six tablespoons regularly. Mix in fruit or vegetable juice, blenderize and drink several glasses of this tonic daily. Add it to baked goods, whole grain cereals. Stir in soup, stews, casseroles. Sprinkle over a raw fruit or vegetable salad. Taken daily, it works almost immediately to regenerate your brain cells, boost nerve-signal transmitter powers and help improve your memory and your entire mental alertness. Give power to your brain with the power vitamin choline, found in lecithin.

THE POWER OIL THAT OPENS UP CHOKED BRAIN CELLS

To promote a better flow of nutrient-carrying oxygen to the choked brain cells, use wheat germ oil as a potent source of Vitamin E which is needed to control the amount of fatty minerals that adhere to the arterial walls leading to the brain. Vitamin E helps to cleanse these walls, promotes a better flow of cell-feeding oxygen to the brain and thereby helps to protect against mental decline or senility.

How to Use Power Vitamin. Use wheat germ oil as part of a salad dressing at least once a day. You could also combine four tablespoons with vegetable juice, blenderize, and drink one or two glasses daily. Use wheat germ oil whenever any fat is required for cooking. You will be giving your bloodstream a high concentration of power Vitamin E which scrubs your brain arteries and helps oxygenate your brain cells to give you power thinking ability.

From "Feebleminded" to "Fantastic" in Five Days

Martha B.J. had so many recurring spells of "forgetfulness" that she faced confinement. At age 71, in otherwise robust good health, this was a sad prospect. Then her attending physician used a power vitamin to help stimulate "sluggish thinking," as he called it. Within five days, this "feebleminded" lady became "fantastic" with her "forever young" thinking abilities. The power vitamin that she takes daily keeps her looking, feeling and acting younger than her granddaughter!

Power Vitamin: Niacin (Vitamin B_3), found in brewer's yeast, ordinary peanut butter, whole grain products offers a unique benefit. It has a vasodilatory (opening up congested blood vessels) action upon the cerebral area to help counteract the effects of brain sclerosis. Taking this power vitamin as a supplement or in the above foods can do much to help you think young at any age!

With the use of these power foods, you can enjoy a dynamic rejuvenation of your thinking components. They help rejuvenate your brain—and the rest of your body, too!

See Circulation, Fatigue, Low Blood Sugar, Weakness.

MOUTH DISORDERS
Power foods that rebuild oral tissues

A healthy mouth can do much to improve the health of your body. When you consider that every bit of nourishing food and drink that you take must first go through your mouth, you realize the importance of having a healthy gateway to the rest of your body.

Nutritional deficiencies as well as general abuse will lower the resistance of your oral tissues to infectious bacteria. Problems of canker sores (wounds and lesions within the mouth and on the tongue), super-sensitivity to temperature of food and liquid, cracked lips, dry mouth, may all be solved with the use of power foods, along with improved living habits.

Basic Program: Eliminate the use of alcohol and tobacco. Harsh chemical irritants in these products will cause erosion of sensitive tissues and give rise to various oral ailments. Avoid the use of harsh seasonings such as salt, pepper, white vinegar, mustard, ketchup. These will irritate and inflame your oral tissues and bring on lesions and disorders. Switch to the use of mild herbs and spices. Eliminate the use of sugar in any form. It tends to devour the B-complex vitamins which are needed to nourish your oral and body membranes. Avoid cola drinks, too, because they contain high amounts of cell-tissue destructive sugar. Twice daily, rinse your mouth with this simple solution: one tablespoon of ordinary baking soda in a glass of warm water. You'll be able to cleanse your mouth and teeth and tongue in a matter of moments. To brush your teeth, use baking soda as a dentifrice. It cleans and disinfects at the same time.

HEAL MOUTH SORES IN FOUR DAYS WITH DELICIOUS POWER FOOD

Troubled with canker sores (blisters) on the inside of her mouth for months, Ida O'T. followed her dentist's advice for speedy relief. Three times a day, after each meal, Ida O'T. would eat a freshly washed apple! She discovered that within four days, the stubborn canker sores were gone. Her whole mouth felt refreshed and clean again. This delicious power food had promoted the healing.

Benefits: A fresh apple, lusciously sweet and naturally juicy, is a treasure of potassium, a mineral that is soothing to irritated skin tissues. The apple also gives a mild fibrous texture and has a natural "detergent" action whereby its pectin content neutralizes the corrosive activities of harmful bacteria. This power food creates an "antiseptic" action in the entire mouth and throat and promotes healing of oral tissues for better health. Eat several freshly washed apples daily for good oral health.

Power Food Mouthwash. To a pint of freshly boiled water, add four tablespoons of apple cider vinegar. Let cool. Then use as a mouthwash. The antiseptic properties of the apple cider vinegar help wash away harmful oral bacteria but do not disturb beneficial bacteria in your mouth and throat.

Strengthening Your Jawbone. Two minerals, calcium and phosphorus, appear to help strengthen the bone matrix of the jaws (and rest of the body) and thereby guard against thinning, also known as osteoporosis. With a strong jawbone, the mouth and oral cavity will be able to resist infectious bacteria. As power minerals, calcium and phosphorus are usually found in similar foods such as yogurt, dairy products and in smaller quantities in carrots, cabbage, kale, broccoli, turnip greens, collards. Eat more of these foods daily to keep your jawbone well nourished.

Problem: About 99 percent of calcium in your body is found in your skeleton. The remaining one percent circulates in your blood and extracellular fluids. If your blood level of calcium should drop, then your blood must "borrow" some of this power mineral from your bones. If taken from your jawbones, then your mouth-oral components start to decline and there is a problem of brittleness and weakness.

Power Food Solution: Have sufficient calcium-phosphorus reserves with the power foods suggested above. Eat one or two cups of yogurt daily. Drink one or two glasses of milk daily. (Skim milk if you are calorie-fat watching.) With adequate amounts of these power food minerals, calcium and phosphorus, your jawbone should be strong and healthy. Your mouth will be healthy, too.

Build a healthier body with a healthier mouth; rebuild your oral tissues and rebuild basic health with the use of everyday power foods.

See Colds, Coughs, "Sweet Tooth."

MUSCULAR ACHES
Power foods that loosen knots and restore youthful flexibility

A muscular ache or cramp is a sudden seizure of a muscle, often so painful that movement is restricted or halted. Muscular aches are often traced to overexertion, loss of body minerals through perspiration, and chronic strain. Constant standing, walking or even sitting may tighten up the muscles, make them feel "knotted" and bring on a pain when trying to change position.

A muscle may be overstretched from a sudden twist of the arm. Taking a wrong step may also cause strain of a muscle that supports the ankle. This will cause aches and spasms in connected body muscles.

Neuritis is another type of muscular ache. A nerve becomes inflamed and this may cause loss of sensation. An abrupt motion may bring on a spasm which is extremely painful.

Your muscles, like other parts of your body, need proper nourishment to help protect against knots and kinks that lead to pain.

THREE POWER FOODS THAT BOOST MUSCLE FLEXIBILITY

Three everyday power foods are high concentrates of nutrients that help create an internal chain reaction to boost muscle flexibility. These are:

1. *Brown Rice.* Contains a powerhouse of manganese, a power mineral that aids in the transmission of impulses between nerve and muscle. Eating a bowl of brown rice will provide a tremendous concentrate of manganese to unlock the knots in your muscles and create soothing relief.
2. *Whole Grain Oatmeal.* A prime source of choline, the power vitamin (along with other muscle-nerve nourishing B-complex vitamins) that is able to help your body produce acetylcholine, the brain neurotransmitter that helps you manipulate your muscles and avoid atrophy.

3. *Orange or Grapefruit.* An excellent source of potassium, the power mineral that works with other nutrients in your extracellular fluids to strongly influence nerve conduction and muscle contractions. Drinking a glass of either (or both) of these power juices will send a much-needed supply of potassium into your bloodstream where this power mineral immediately helps soothe muscular tightness, loosen knots, and make your entire body more youthfully flexible.

POWER FOOD PROGRAM FOR YOUNG MUSCLES

Start off your day with speedy energy. Have a breakfast consisting of steamed brown rice, a bowl of whole grain oatmeal (made with milk for calcium boosting) and a glass of orange-grapefruit juice combination. You will be providing your body with powerful manganese, choline, potassium, three power minerals that act as muscle rejuvenators . . . in a matter of moments. You'll enjoy an ache-free working day.

THE HEALING POWER OF WATER

Drinking lots of water daily helps moisture and lubricate your cells and tissues (your muscles are actually bundles of fibers consisting of cells and tissues) to prevent irritation and chafing. As a power food, water is an all-natural muscle rejuvenator.

For any muscle ache, use external water in the form of contrasting hot-cold compresses. Soak yourself in a tepid tub of water and your muscular aches will subside. You'll emerge with more flexibility and youthful health.

THE POWER MINERAL THAT WASHES AWAY MUSCLE ACHES

What Causes Muscle Ache? Use of your muscles, even if mild, will cause an outpouring of a substance known as lactic acid. This is a normal metabolic product of glucose metabolism. When the lactic acid accumulates, the end feeling is that of fatigue. This is nature's way of telling you to stop and rest. A problem is that too high a level of lactic acid because of excessive glucose reaction may cause an aching feeling. This may be mild or severe, depending upon the individual's tolerance of this metabolic product. But a muscle aches because lactic acid is irritating the cells, tissues and fibers.

How Can Power Mineral Ease-Erase Ache? Calcium is a power mineral that helps control excessive lactic acid accumulation by *diluting* and *neutralizing* it. When you ingest this power mineral, calcium goes to work immediately to inhibit the lactic acid's effect on your neuromuscular system. This power mineral coats the ends of your nerve cells (called synapses) and establishes communication and electrical connections between nerve cells. Therefore, this power mineral combines with lactic acid around the sensitive nerve endings. Calcium prevents the lactic acid from irritating the nervous system. This power mineral must be available at all times in adequate amounts to shield your nerve cells from lactic acid irritation.

How Can This Power Mineral Be Made Abundantly Available? Plan to drink several glasses of milk daily (skim milk for less fat and calories). Enjoy yogurt, too. Cheeses are good sources of calcium. Health stores and pharmacies have calcium supplements available. Increase your intake of calcium and your muscles and nerves will soon be "untied" and you'll discover greater flexibility and youthful agility.

Loosen up muscular congestion with power foods and you'll open up your potential for rejuvenated flexibility.

See Arthritis, Bachache, Leg and Foot Problems, Stiffness.

NAUSEA
Power foods that correct upset stomach

Nausea is a condition in which there is a regurgitation of foods and liquids. It is common with viral infections (not necessarily with a fever) of the digestive tract. Nausea is also a reaction to certain medications or as a result of eating foods which are contaminated or which disagree with your digestive tract. Emotional stress, eating hurriedly, combining the wrong types of foods may also bring on a nausea attack.

Each bout with nausea causes a loss of important nutrients to your body. Furthermore, nausea may also cause such a serious drain on your resources that your body system risks being undernourished and developing various ailments. Nausea is a breakdown of your body's defenses against infectious bacteria. To help you maintain resistance to outside virus and other harmful elements, to build a strong barrier against illness, protect yourself against nausea with power food programs.

POWER FOOD BEVERAGES FOR MINERAL FORTIFICATION

Dehydration calls for speedy use of various power food beverages. The use of fruit and vegetable juices will help replace the minerals that have been lost in nausea. Extreme thirst and dryness of the mouth and tongue suggest the need for mineral replacement through these various juices.

Power Program: Replenish your chafing and burning digestive and oral tissues with cooling minerals from fruit juices such as apple, berry, pineapple, pear, peach, papaya, or grape, either singly or in combination. Vegetable juices that are digestive-soothing include carrot, cucumber, lettuce, cabbage, tomato, and green pepper, either singly or in combination. To help control stomach churning, just *sip slowly* of a room-temperature beverage of your choice. You should be able to help replenish your parched and thirsty digestive tissues and replace the delicate electrolyte balance in your bloodstream with these power juices so that nausea will be eased and controlled within a few hours.

Soothe, Pamper, Content Digestive System. When nausea occurs, avoid solid foods. Sit up or lie down, but keep your upper body partly *raised* to avoid backup of ingested foods that may increase nausea. If nothing stays down, suck on ice chips. This seems to ease stomach rumbling. Loosen tight clothing. Apply soothing-healing warmth to your stomach in the form of a heating pad or a hot water bag. If you feel chilled, cover yourself with a warm robe or blanket. You might wrap a woolen scarf around your waistline to induce further pampering warmth. Avoid any emotional or physical stress. These home helps soothe and relax your upset stomach and help heal nausea in a few hours, or sooner.

Cucumbers: Power Mineral Food for Nausea Relief. Folklore healers suggest the use of peeled cucumbers to help heal nausea in a short while. This vegetable is a prime source of such minerals as sulfur, magnesium and manganese which appear to soothe and cool that burning sensation that reacts in nausea. Eating a plate of cucumber slices will help send healing minerals to your frazzled digestive tract and calm down flutter-causing nausea.

Power Grain to Correct Nausea. Ordinary barley is a power source of polyunsaturated fatty acids and mucilaginous ingredients that help to moisturize the digestive organs and will create a *protective coating action* on these organs to soothe and correct nausea unrest. To recover from nausea quickly, simply prepare a bowl of barley, flavor with a bit of honey, and eat slowly. Within minutes, this power grain will help regenerate the irritated digestive organs and provide soothing relief and correction of nausea.

Power Tea for Swift Relief. Golden seal herb tea (from health store or pharmacy) contains minerals from the deep rooted soil which are able to heal and soothe the distress of an upset stomach. Just brew several cups of golden seal herb tea, flavor with lemon juice and honey, and sip slowly to help create a "tranquil stomach" within a few moments. Nausea reactions will be relieved and the drain on vital nutrients will be halted.

Folklore Healers. Raspberry leaf tea is believed to soothe an outraged digestive system and bring swift nausea relief. Eating wild raspberries is also helpful. Chewing on ginger sticks and drinking ginger tea offers soothing relief.

Bitter Fruits for Speedy Relief. You'll enjoy speedy relief with bitter fruits. These are power healers that work almost at once.

Chew and then swallow any grated citrus peel (freshly washed and scrubbed before use). Grate the rind of a lemon or lime, add a little grated carrot to make it more palatable, then chew and eat with a spoon. This tart, spicy and almost bitter flavor appears to create healing of the outraged digestive system in a few minutes.

With the use of improved living habits and power foods, you should be able to build a barrier of resistance against infection by controlling and healing nausea in a short time.

See CRAMPS, DIGESTIVE DISTURBANCES.

NECK PAINS
Power foods that melt away tight spots

Neck pains occur when you keep your head in one position for an extended length of time. In your neck are muscles which are composed of many separate fibers. They tend to contract when subjected to a stationary position and this causes a form of pain. Neck bones are also subjected to this strain. These bones are covered by periosteum, a strong fibrous membrane. When your head is kept rigid, there is a form of congestion so that the blood supply to the bone is unable to get through the periosteum. This leads to a form of malnutrition in this region and your neck muscles and bone react by causing a form of pain.

Stress and tension, whether emotional or physical (or both), may also induce a muscular-bone congestion and a reactive pain. Sudden shock will also cause a stiffening of these neck muscles and pain results.

In whiplash, a neck injury occurs, usually in a vehicle accident in which the car is hit from the rear, or else is forced to make a sudden swerve or halt. The head is snapped back, then forward, like a whip. An injury occurs in the lower level of the neck vertebra where the muscles and ligaments are strained or torn. Whiplash neck pain may also be caused when you land sharply or suddenly on your feet or buttocks.

To help melt away these tight spots and enjoy freedom from neck pain, use power foods to bolster healing as well as resistance to this disorder.

THE POWER FRUIT FAST THAT HEALED NECK PAINS

Oscar McG. suffered severe neck pains and incapacitating whiplash when he had to make a sudden turn on the highway to avoid being struck by an oncoming truck. The jarring sensation caused him to instinctively stiffen his body and shoulders, and he suffered agonizing pains in the back of his neck as a result. Oscar McG. tried medications which gave him so many side effects that they were worse than his neck pains!

His osteopathic physician recommended the use of a high-powered mineral that would be able to promote swift and thorough healing of the strained and shocked nerve-muscle-bone network in his neck. Oscar McG. was put on a three-day fruit fast. By the end of this time, his neck pains were gone. He felt completely healed. He felt younger than young again, thanks to the high-powered mineral in the fruit fast.

Basic Neck-Healing Program: For three days, take nothing but potassium-rich fruits of all kinds. Drink their juices, too. No other food. These fruits are prunes, dates, figs, bananas, oranges, grapefruits, tangerines, grapes, pineapple, apricots, peaches. You may eat them as part of a salad or individually, as you prefer. You may drink their juices either singly or in any desired combination.

Power Healing Benefits: The power of potassium is able to work without digestive interference of other nutrients, therefore the benefit of this special fast. Potassium helps to nourish the aching fibers which make up your neck muscles. Potassium is also able to enervate your bloodstream to send a supply of important nourishment through the periosteum and right into the bone where healing is speedily and effectively created. Neck muscle cramps are soothed with the potassium contained in these fruits and their juices. It is the most abundant body mineral, next to calcium, and helps regulate important pain-relieving balance between the intra- and extracellular fluids in the tissues of your neck muscles. This power mineral works very swiftly to give welcome relief from neck pain. It improves total body health, too.

Hot Water Pack Is Soothing. The use of hot water is beneficial because the warmth will relax the strained muscles and provide soothing comfort. Water is a power food whether taken internally or used externally. Just apply a comfortably hot compress to the nape of your neck. Let remain until cool, then apply a fresh hot compress. Thirty minutes of this hot water pack will do much to promote swift healing.

Silk Scarf Is Folklore Healer. Wrap a silk scarf or cloth around your neck. Let it remain as long as possible. Wear it all day. Sleep with it on.

Benefit: Folklorists say that the silk seals in body heat to exert muscle-relaxing warmth. The silk-induced warmth improves the sluggish blood flow to the fibrous membranes where nourishment will help ease and dispose of the pain.

Power Liniment. Dissolve one-third teaspoon of dry camphor and one-third teaspoon of dry mustard in one pint of apple cider vinegar. Now add one pint of wheat germ oil and one pint of rubbing alcohol. Shake or blenderize until thoroughly combined. Use this power liniment upon the aching portion of your neck. Massage gently. Let your skin absorb as much as possible. Cover with a flannel or woolen cloth. Let remain overnight.

Benefits: Potassium and other minerals become invigorated by the warmth of the dry mustard and also stimulated by the minerals in the other ingredients. You'll feel a relaxing muscular warmth seep through the nape of your neck almost in moments. Overnight, your neck pain should be gone. You'll awaken with the feeling that you have a brand new body!

Melt away tight spots and enjoy a flexible and youthful neck (and body) with the aid of power foods.

See BACKACHE, HEADACHES, MUSCULAR ACHES, SPINAL COLUMN, STIFFNESS.

NERVOUSNESS
Power foods that calm anxiety and soothe neuritis

Nervousness, also known as neuritis, is an inflammation of a nerve or nerves anywhere in the body. This irritation may be caused by emotional or physical unrest or a combination of the two. Since your body has millions of pain, pressure and hearing receptors, just one upset will cause a neuritis attack.

The parts of your body you commonly call nerves are really bundles of nerve fibers, some so thin that a bundle an inch thick may contain 25,000 fibers. In several parts of your body, nerve fibers branch out and connect with other nerve bundles. This makes up an entire network from head to toe so that you are, in fact, ruled by your nervous system.

Body Upset Causes Neuritis. Nerve inflammation (polyneuritis) is often caused by a mechanical injury such as pressure on a nerve while sleeping, prolonged cramped position, constantly bending down or maintaining a congested posture, and violent overexertion. A vascular ailment such as a constricted artery will bring on a neuritis attack. A nutritional deficiency of the B-complex vitamins (especially nerve-nourishing thiamine or Vitamin B_1) or of minerals will also assault the delicate nerve fiber mechanism and trigger distress signals. Avoid or correct these body upset conditions and you are less likely to develop nervousness in most of its painful forms. To shield yourself against nervousness, use power foods to raise your levels of resistance and help you enjoy better health and longer pain-free years of happier living.

POWER FOOD RECIPE FOR SPEEDY RELAXATION OF "CRYING" NERVES

Rose F. L. would cry out in agonizing pain whenever she was stricken with neuritis. Her shoulder felt inflamed. Often the pain would spread until the right side of her body felt like one massive ache. Rose F.L. had tried various medications which numbed the pain, but when the effect wore off, she suffered all the more. She often lamented that her nerves were "crying" with pain. So was she!

Her neurologist suggested that she try a simple and tasty nutritious recipe which consisted of two everyday foods. In combination, these two foods offered *two* basic ingredients (along with other healers) that would combine to help soothe and relax her "crying" nerves and bring speedy relaxation.

Rose F.L. followed the program. In a bowl, she would pour skim milk and then add a cup of whole grain granola cereal. For added effect, she used several tablespoons of wheat germ. Rose F.L. ate this cereal in the morning. Within an hour, the throbbing pain subsided. The inflammation cooled off. Her shoulder and right side felt more flexible. Before the next hour was over, the neuritis-nervousness syndrome was gone! Now Rose F.L. enjoys this power recipe almost daily and is free from the stubborn pain-causing nervousness.

Benefits: The milk is a power source of calcium, a mineral that combines with the energy-producing powers of Vitamin B_1 of the granola and wheat germ to help coat the raw nerve endings so that they are not subjected to hurtful abrasiveness and will not "cry" out with body-producing pain. Calcium unites with Vitamin B_1 to cause better nerve-muscle contractibility, to create a shift to adrenalin-like neuro-humors (nerve segments) to help relieve pressure and pain. In effect, this simple power food recipe, using two or three power ingredients, creates balm to soothe frazzled nerves and calm down anxiety.

Correct Sleeping Position for Better Nerve Nourishment. If you put pressure on any limb while sleeping, you squeeze the nerves, and this causes blood congestion. This backup will lead to nervousness as well as to pain in the particular region. Pressures on your arm and shoulder will disturb the lubricating system; this upsets the delicate sac in the shoulder joint which should be moistened by a nutrient-carrying oily fluid. A breakdown of this moisturizing system because of sleeping pressure will trigger neuritis. Train yourself *not* to sleep on your side. Avoid any prolonged pressure—whether sleeping, standing, sitting, walking or running. When this pressure error is corrected, your lubricating system functions healthfully and your better-nourished nerves are relieved of pain.

POWER FOOD REMEDIES FOR NERVOUSNESS

Warm Water. You soak in it for at least 20 minutes a night. The action of the water against your skin will soothe your nerves and help you calm down in body and mind.

Dill Tea. Herbal healers suggest using dill tea because it contains a soporific that is a tonic to your nerves. Just add one teaspoon of dill to one cup of freshly boiled water. Flavor with lemon juice and honey. Two cups a day will help ease nerve pressure.

Kelp Instead of Table Salt. This seaweed product is a powerhouse of concentrated calcium, phosphorus, potassium, choline and many other trace elements that nourish your nerve endings. Use it as a replacement for table salt, which is abrasive and irritating and tends to chafe and erode the myalin sheath (nerve covering) to expose the raw fibers beneath and create serious pain. A simple change to kelp as a flavoring instead of salt will do much to protect you from physical and mental nervousness.

THE POWER MINERAL FOR FREEDOM FROM NERVOUSNESS

Manganese, an essential trace mineral, has power to help you enjoy freedom from nervousness. This power mineral stimulates the *adenylate cyclase activity* in your brain and related nerve-muscle tissues in the rest of your body. It is this activity that regulates the action of important brain neurotransmitters. This in turn soothes the nerve fibers. The ACA action "tells" the nerves to rest, and this helps free you from nervousness and physical pain. This is made possible through this power mineral, manganese.

Sources of Power Mineral: Whole grain breads, cereals, nuts, seeds, leafy vegetables. *Suggestion:* For speedy ACA reaction and healing of neuritis, have a handful of shelled sunflower, squash or pumpkin seeds with you. Munch on them regularly. You'll be sending a high concentration of nerve-soothing manganese into your system. You'll alert the ACA process so your brain will say "be calm" to your nerves. You'll feel "glad all over" in a short time.

Calm down anxiety, cool off your inflamed nerves, sooth your mind and body with the use of tasty power foods you can enjoy anytime, almost anywhere. They work within minutes!

See FATIGUE, ITCHING, TREMBLING.

PROSTATE
Power foods that keep the male gland youthfully healthy

The prostate is often called the gland of youth because its hormones help keep the male feeling alert and active and filled with the joy of life. Keep the prostate nourished with power foods and it will help keep the male feeling invigorated and responsive to daily obligations.

The prostate is located just below the bladder and encircling the urethra where it exits from the bladder. It secretes a part of the seminal fluid in which sperm from the testes are suspended. If there is a problem with the prostate, then the release of various hormones is restricted and this may lead to ill health as well as premature aging.

In *prostatitis,* inflammation of the urethra (the tube that carries urine from the bladder through the penis) may become chronic and cause stricture (closing). This may block free passage of urine. In an *enlarged prostate,* urine is blocked from passage and collects in the bladder. This may have dire consequences, causing kidney or bladder stones, organ inflammation and uremia. To keep the prostate gland healthy is to keep the entire body filled with vim and vigor.

Youth-Building Benefits of Healthy Prostate. Prostate hormones are sent into the bloodstream to help create a feeling of energy, skin health, emotional vitality, better physical abilities. Prostate hormones influence the vigor of body organs to create a feeling of total youth, even in advancing years. Prostate hormones may well be considered man's internal "fountain of youth." Keep the springs flowing through your bloodstream and you will continue to feel the joy of youthful life.

THE POWER FOOD THAT STRENGTHENS THE PROSTATE

Prostate hormones contain a large supply of a little-known power food element—zinc. This trace mineral has an energizing effect upon the often sluggish prostate gland and causes it to become better activated to release more of its *testosterone* hormone, the rejuvenating fluid that helps to revive the entire body. Zinc is the energizing factor that promotes testosterone release and distribution so that it can help strengthen the prostate and related organs and boost male vigor.

Sources of Prostate-Strengthening Power Food: Herring, beef, milk, wheat bran, whole grain oatmeal, wheat germ, peas, carrots. Zinc is also available as a supplement from health stores and pharmacies. *Suggestion:* Plan to use the whole grains daily. Enjoy the vegetables. Use herring as part of a main dish, together with peas, carrots and other vegetables. Lean beef will give you good zinc supplies. You will be strengthening your prostate with this power food mineral, and helping yourself enjoy more youthful years of vitality-filled health.

The Power Food That Ended "Getting Up at Night" in Four Days. Earl W. was troubled with having to keep "getting up at night" for bathroom trips. A nutritionally starved prostate creates the desire for frequent urination. Not only did this disturb Earl W.'s sleep, but it weakened him so that he started to look haggard. Although only in his middle 60's, he started to shuffle with a stooped gait that made him look much older. His urologist said that in order to supply the proper nutrition for his prostate, he should try one simple but powerful food that would help correct the problem. Earl W. had to eat about a pound of shelled pumpkin seeds daily. He could also use shelled sunflower seeds. Earl W. followed this simple power food program. Within two days, he perked up, looked youthful, and walked with flexible agility. Within four days, he no longer had to get up nightly. He enjoyed healthy sleep. Now he looked much younger. He felt young, too. Now he eats pumpkin and sunflower seeds daily. He calls them his "youth food" because they revived his sluggish prostate gland. All this in just four days!

Benefit: Pumpkin and sunflower seeds are high concentrated sources of polyunsaturated fatty acids together with Vitamin E as well as the most important phosphorus, iron, Vitamins A and B-complex and other nutrients. But the fatty acids and Vitamin E have a powerhouse effect of correcting prostate gland disorders. These power nutrients stimulate the gland to release more testosterone and help open up blocked ducts to allow a free release of urine. They correct "backup" congestion through this method. These simple, tasty seeds are power foods that help keep your prostate (and body) feeling and looking "forever young."

Herbal Power Tonics. Brew a tea from such herbs as buchu leaves, bearberry, cubeb berries, saw palmetto. Use individually or in combination. These herbs appear to soothe an irritated prostate-bladder condition, help correct structural damage, cool inflammation. They contain plant proteins which appear to strengthen the muscles of the prostate-urethral network so that there is less incontinence. These herbs are available at most health stores as well as herbal pharmacies. Use them regularly. They will help soothe prostate irregularities and bolster the function of this all-important male youth gland.

With the help of easily available power foods, you should be able to easily keep your male gland youthfully healthy. Your entire body will radiate the glow of youth when your prostate is nourished with power foods.

See Sex-Related Disorders, Sexual Powers.

SEX-RELATED DISORDERS
Power foods that ease male/female "change of life" reactions

In men, a change of life also occurs in the middle years. Body responses may become a bit slower. The network of endocrine glands undergoes certain changes. Metabolism is adjusted so that the less active man will be able to enjoy life without the large amount of internal activity that is important in the very young years.

It is nature's way of helping the body adjust to changes in living habits.

Because there is a slight readjustment of the gland-hormone rhythm, the male may experience some difficulties at the outset. Known as the "male climacteric," this condition may make the male feel inadequate. This is only a temporary feeling. It is important to help balance your hormonal release and keep your body invigorated to meet the responsibilities of the middle years. This is done with the use of power foods that not only ease the male change of life reactions but also help him become vigorous and healthy even in later years.

In women, the menopause ("change of life") is the cessation of menstruation; it results in a cessation of the female hormones. While the body must adjust to lesser supplies, the woman can continue to enjoy vigorous good health and youthful responses with the use of body-nourishing power foods.

Symptoms: In male and female, symptoms usually include a feeling of excessive warmth (similar to a fever), chills, tingling, frequent urination, fatigue, giddiness, blood pressure rise, appetite irregularities, nervous irritability, emotional instability, crying jags, bouts of anxiety and moodiness.

POWER FOODS THAT BOOST NATURAL HORMONE PRODUCTION

Taking up the slack of the sluggish male and female glands, power foods are able to help boost natural hormone production. These power foods energize the metabolic system so that there is a corresponding release of hormones to supplement those that have been diminished.

Licorice Water: European Power Beverage. In many European countries, especially France where the people seem to be ageless and forever romantic, the change of life is eliminated with the use of a simple power food—*Licorice Water!* To prepare, just mix one teaspoon of powdered licorice (from health stores or herbalists) in a glass of natural club soda. You now have a powerhouse of nutrition because the licorice contains substances equal to that of male and female hormones. It may even be considered a "hormone tonic" from nature. Drink one or two freshly prepared glasses of *Licorice Water* daily. The plant hormones revive the sluggish glands and tend to release important substances that will create a feeling of vigor and youthfulness so that there is no change of life reaction. It is the French way to perpetual youth!

Sarsaparilla Root. This herb contains botanical forms of *testosterone* together with *epitestosterone* and *androstenedione*, male hormones that help revive the entire body. When brewed as a tea, sarsaparilla root will nourish the hormone-making ducts of the male gland and promote a feeling of energy and vigor. It is the tasty way to help enjoy a total extension of the prime of life.

Youth Secret from the Orient. For thousands of years, the ageless Orientals (who are known for becoming parents even in their late years) have relied upon a power food herb that is said to energize the body and create Tibet-like eternal youth. *Ginseng* is the name of this Oriental herb which has remained secret until relatively recent times. The ginseng root, shaped like a man, is said to have a tonic effect; it contains natural stimulants that tend to activate the glands to release ample amounts of youth-restoring hormones. *Ginseng has the power to supplement and even substitute for hormones that body glands no longer release.*

How to Use Power Herb: At any health store or pharmacy, obtain ginseng root. Eat a little piece every day. Chew well. You'll be giving your glands and your other body organs a supercharged feeling with the highly concentrated forces in this Oriental youth secret. Ginseng tea is also available and should be used regularly. Nourish your body with ginseng and you will be rewarded with a new lease on life.

THE POWER VEGETABLE WITH YOUTH-BUILDING POWERS

The simple *onion* may well hold the secret of better health and longer life through glandular rejuvenation in the middle years for men and women.

Power Benefit: European electrobiologists and gerontologists (specialists in prolonging health in older people) have discovered that the onion releases an ultraviolet emission called *mitogenic radiation* or M rays. These natural electrified radiations tend to stimulate cellular activity and thereby promote the rejuvenation of the entire system. In particular, the onion, as a power food, contains *allicepum*, a substance that boosts body circulation, strengthens the activities of most body organs and creates a feeling of youthfulness in older people. This common vegetable is a power food that may well be the sought-after secret of perpetual youth.

Suggestion: Use onions either raw or cooked for salads, soups, stews, casseroles, baked dishes and wherever a flavoring agent is needed. Plan to eat onions daily. This power food may help you enjoy many years of vigorous health, regardless of your age.

For any sex-related disorders of the change of life, the use of power foods will help ease reactions and then help you enjoy the second half of your life—with double vigor!

See PROSTATE, SEXUAL POWERS.

SEXUAL POWERS
Power foods that rejuvenate youth glands

Your marital vigor is influenced by the foods you eat. In particular, your endocrine and sex glands are biological laboratories which need power foods in order to influence the healthy function of your youth glands as well as the organs involved in lovemaking. The quality of nutrition influences the state of sexual health.

Your glands are directly responsible for sexual activity. Most of your body's functions are influenced by these glands. When you nourish your youth glands with power foods, they are able to release an abundant supply of hormones and other secretions that energize, invigorate and activate more than just your libidinal impulses, but your general well-being, emotional and physical, as well.

To help rejuvenate your youth glands, nourish them with power foods and they will reward you with healthy sexual powers during your lifetime.

THE POWER FOOD THAT WARMS UP MARITAL COLDNESS

A trace element, zinc, is a power food that is able to supercharge the endocrine gland network and create a rich release of hormones that can warm up the entire body and melt so-called marital coldness.

Youth Power of Zinc. This power mineral reportedly is able to energize the sex glands to help cause maturity of the reproductive organs, boost sperm motility, decrease prostatitis and normalize hormone release, and replace the zinc loss occasioned by excessive prostate secretion. The prostate and prostatic secretions in males and the normal ova in females are high in zinc, attesting to the importance of this power mineral for healthy youth glands. A zinc deficiency will lead to partial atrophy of the sex-influencing glands and to premature aging. It is zinc that dispatches an enzyme known as *acid phosphatase* to influence a healthy libidinal drive in both male and female through glandular activation. Zinc may well be the scientific aphrodisiac long sought for to prolong the sexual prime of life.

Sources of Power Food: Herring, milk, beef, beef liver, peas, whole grains. *Suggestions:* Plan to eat herring several times weekly. Also include a zinc food supplement (health stores or pharmacies) daily. You will be reviving, regenerating and rejuvenating your glands so that you will be able to enjoy a healthy libidinal response.

Power Seeds for Power Sex. Shelled pumpkin and sunflower seeds are highly concentrazed sources of zinc. When you eat these power seeds, you release the important mineral that influences hormone production. Eating several cups of seeds daily will do much to keep your glands functioning actively to help you enjoy power sex.

THE MIDDLE EASTERN POWER FOOD FOR YOUTHFUL VIRILITY

Sesame, cultivated for thousands of years, is often named in ancient Middle Eastern and Oriental writings as a powerful virility food. Middle Easterners use it regularly, especially in the form of *halvah,* which is a mixture of sesame and honey. The "forever young, forever virile" people of ancient Babylonia used it to enhance their sexual appeal. Today, sesame may be used in seed form, in oil, in a butter-like spread called *tahini*. It is considered a gland-rejuvenating power food that boosts youthful virility at all ages.

Benefits: Sesame is a highly concentrated source of lecithin, the phosphorized fatty substance that is an essential component of hormones, especially those of the male. Lecithin, from sesame, is able to energize the master pituitary gland to release hormones that serve to revitalize the entire body and create a healthy desire for libidinal fulfillment. Also in sesame is a high supply of magnesium together with potassium, which help erase "tiredness" and create a feeling of youthful desire in male and female. This ancient Middle Eastern and Oriental food is recognized today as an important power food for healthy lovemaking.

From "Bedroom Coldness" to "Bridal Warmth" in Three Days. Anna O'N. felt deprived because she could not respond to her husband's desire for affection. She sobbed when he called her "cold" and said she made him feel old and useless. They were drawing apart. Seeking help from an endocrinologist, Anna O'N was told to follow a nutritional improvement program. Both she and her husband were to take zinc supplements, then to boost their intake of lecithin through sesame seeds. She was advised to eat *halvah*. Not only was this Middle Eastern "aphrodisiac" delicious to taste, but it contained, according to modern science, a high concentration of zinc, lecithin, magnesium and potassium. This combination would revitalize sluggish glands. She was told to eat pumpkin and sunflower seeds for more nutritional revitalization. Following this program, both Anna O'N. and her husband so rejuvenated themselves that they went from "bedroom coldness" to "bridal warmth" within three days! They call the halvah and seeds and supplements their "love foods"!

POWER TONIC FOR GLAND REJUVENATION

1½ glasses of skim milk
2 tablespoons brewer's yeast
2 egg yolks (optional, if cholesterol-watching)
2 tablespoons honey
1 tablespoon sesame seed oil
2 tablespoons bran
2 tablespoons sesame seeds
2 tablespoons shelled pumpkin seeds
2 tablespoons shelled sunflower seeds
2 teaspoons lecithin granules
1 tablespoon crushed ice

Combine all ingredients and blenderize for just two minutes or until fully combined, when seeds are liquefied. Sip slowly. Enjoy the taste.

Benefits: Within minutes, the high zinc content of this *Power Tonic* will revitalize your glands to boost better hormone secretion and a healthier desire for lovemaking. The high mineral-vitamin-protein combo of the power foods in the *tonic* will supercharge your body for speedy response. Enjoy this *Power Tonic* several hours before a romance and you will discover new youth and healthy fulfillment.

With the helpful use of power foods, you can reach the peak of your sexual energy and remain there for a long, long time.

See PROSTATE, SEX-RELATED DISORDERS.

SINUSITIS
Power foods that relieve congestion and restore better breathing

The sinuses are air spaces that empty their secretions into the nasal cavity through narrow ducts. This drainage method is not always efficient. The ducts are so situated that you would need to stand on your head to facilitate proper drainage. But you do need healthy sinuses. They act as the resonating chambers for your voice. They also serve to warm and liquefy the air you breathe. They are an integral part of your nasal filtering system. Air within your sinus openings helps reduce the weight of your skull. If an excess of fluid or toxic wastes accumulates in this air space, you develop headaches and problems of what is called sinusitis.

In this condition, there is nasal blockage. In addition to a stuffed nose, there is headache, usually frontal or periorbital (around the eye), regardless of which sinuses are congested. In more acute sinusitis, there may be fever, mental sluggishness, chills, even dizziness. If neglected, sinusitis lingers on and on and may worsen with each attack. It is nature's way of telling you to correct errors to allow improved breathing, better health, more vitality through blood-enriched oxygen.

Basic Suggestions: Eliminate tobacco and alcohol. They introduce toxic wastes into the cells and mucous membranes of the nasal passages. Avoid foods and beverages that are too cold because the chill forces nasal passages to tighten up and this may trigger off a sinusitis attack. Replace strong spices such as salt, pepper, mustard, ketchup with more natural herbs as flavorings. Keep yourself dry when going outdoors. Body chill provokes a sinusitis attack. Rapid changes in barometric pressure (as in airplane flights) tend to injure the membranes lining the sinuses. Protect yourself against all of these things for greater immunity against sinusitis.

THE POWER VITAMIN THAT DEFENDS AGAINST SINUS ATTACKS

Vitamin A is a powerful nutrient that is able to boost natural defense and even healing of sinus attacks. This power vitamin nourishes the mucous membranes and the hair-like cilia lining the sinuses. The tiny cilia hairs brush the mucus forward with a *metachronical* method. That is, the cilia propel the mucus forward to the next row of cilia, which then take up this process. Like ocean waves or fields of grain, the cilia hairs work together to keep the mucous flow moving. Vitamin A boosts this *metachronical* process to protect against backup or congestion.

A Vitamin A deficiency may cause the tiny cilia hairs to become broken, destroyed and thinned out. The mucus becomes locked in, unable to be *metachronically* removed. This gives rise to sinusitis.

Vitamin A Sources: Broccoli, chard, collards, kale, turnip greens, watercress, carrots, pumpkin, sweet potatoes, winter squash, apricots, cantaloupes, mangoes, persimmons, tomatoes, liver, kidneys, fish liver oils, fortified dairy products, Cheddar cheese.

Sinus Healing Power Elixir: Blenderize carrots, apricots, tomatoes to create an elixir that is a powerhouse of Vitamin A, the essential cilia-strengthening nutrient. This elixir will help build resistance to recurring sinus attacks.

POWER FOLK REMEDIES

Build resistance to sinus attacks, relieve congestion and restore better and move youthful breathing with these power folk remedies that use items available in your cupboard, local food store, health store or pharmacy.

- *Cod Liver Oil.* A prime source of membrane-healing Vitamin A. Take several tablespoons daily. Mix with fruit juice for more palatability.
- *Vegetable Remedy.* Mix together chopped onions and garlic. Add parsley to neutralize the strong odor of these vegetables. Chew thoroughly. Eat a portion daily. Strong volatile oils in these vegetables soothe the mucous lining of the nose and sinuses, help to detoxify potentially harmful bacteria.
- *Food Remedy.* Carrots, cucumbers, blueberries contain power-packed nutrients that can build a barrier against recurring sinus attacks. They also help unblock stuffy noses. Eat these fresh or juiced, singly or in combination.
- *Horseradish-Lemon Sauce.* Mix grated horseradish and freshly squeezed lemon juice until you have a thick sauce. Take one tablespoon of this sauce in the morning and another in the evening. Do *not* eat or drink anything for one hour before or after taking this remedy. It helps clear up the most stubborn nasal congestion.

- *Herbal Healer.* From an herbal pharmacist, obtain horehound leaves and roots. Boil one teaspoon herb to one cup boiling water until you have a thick syrup. Take one tablespoon of this syrup daily. It will help clear up your sinus condition within two or three days at the most.

With better body care and the use of power foods, you should be able to relieve congestion, breathe better, feel better all over.

See ALLERGIES, ASTHMA, BREATHING DIFFICULTIES, COLDS.

SKIN
Power foods that rejuvenate your body envelope

Your skin is your largest body envelope. You have over 3000 square inches of surface area. Your skin weighs about six pounds, is twice as heavy as your brain and liver. Your skin receives one-third of all the blood circulating throughout your body. This body envelope has more functions than just covering you up. It protects your tissues, organs and bones; acts as a thermostat, a waste disposal unit, a defensive wall against bacterial invasion. Your skin is also a storehouse for fats and essential nutrients.

Young Skin = Better Health, Longer Life. The youthful appearance of your skin is considered a barometer of your basic health and life span. Since your skin absorbs the first abuses from the outside environment, it often falls victim to disorders such as blemishes, dark spots, wrinkling, premature aging, more serious ailments that are symptomatic of metabolic errors within your body. A young skin, with the use of power foods, is your ticket to a journey through life with youthful health.

POWER FOODS, HOME REMEDIES, SKIN-REJUVENATING PROGRAMS

Through the ages, certain power foods from garden and kitchen turn up over and over again as skin-rejuvenating aids—eggs, honey, milk, oatmeal, bran, cucumber, oil. Let's see how these power foods and home remedies can help rejuvenate your skin, often in a few minutes.

- *Egg White.* Clean your face well. Rub with egg white. This power food will tighten on your skin. Let remain 30 minutes. Splash off. Your complexion now looks rosy, glowing, immaculate.
- *Paste Masque.* Make a paste of oatmeal or cornmeal by mixing with a little water. Spread on your face and let remain 20 minutes. Splash off with warm and then cool water. Blemishes lighten and the skin firms up. Wrinkles appear to flatten out, too.
- *Avocado Paste.* Mash the green avocado "meat" and apply to your face. Let remain 20 minutes. Splash off with warm and cool water. Helps take off grime; removes stubborn dirt that clogs the pores; helps to heal blemishes.
- *Fruit Juice.* To refresh tired eyelids, soak gauze in orange juice and apply to your eyelids. Apply to the rest of your face, if desired. Keep the gauze wet with orange juice. Keep re-applying. Let remain 30 minutes, then splash off. Your skin will glow; your eyelids will look nice and youthful.
- *Cucumber Wash.* Mash some cut-up cucumber in cool water. Now spread all over your skin. Minerals help nourish your skin and ease or erase lines and creases. After 30 minutes, splash off.
- *Dry Skin Lotion.* Rub your face lightly with olive oil. The polyunsaturated fatty acids nourish the reservoirs beneath surface to create healthy and youthful moisture, the key to better skin appearance. Let remain an hour. Then splash off with warm and cool water.
- *Melon Masque.* An ancient skin-rejuvenating remedy is to mash a honeydew melon and use the pulp as a masque. Or mix the mashed melon with ordinary petroleum jelly and spread on your face. This helps fortify natural moisture to soften wrinkles and crease lines.
- *Pretty Hands.* Rub with salt, lemon wedge or raw potato after doing dishwashing or other skin-chafing work.

- *Soften Elbows.* Just rest each rough or red elbow in half a grapefruit while you are reading.
- *Soften Feet.* Rub in ordinary cooking oil on calluses, heels or rough spots on your feet. Slip on clean socks. Let remain overnight. Next morning, wash off. Repeat regularly for softer feet.
- *Smooth Away Chafed Skin.* Wet oatmeal to a paste consistency. Rub wherever you have chafed skin. Keep rubbing. Let remain ten minutes, then splash off. After doing this once or twice you'll have softer and younger looking skin.

A YOUTHFUL SKIN IS AN INSIDE JOB

Power foods nourish from within your body to create a healthy metabolism and cleansing system so that your skin will glow with youthful health.

Daily, plan to eat lots of fresh fruits and vegetables and their juices. They offer you high concentrates of skin-nourishing vitamins, minerals, enzymes. Include whole grains for polyunsaturated fatty acids and roughage so that you are able to enjoy regularity. Internal cleanliness helps to give you external health. Nourish your skin with amino acids from protein foods such as lean meats, poultry, dairy products, seeds, peas, beans, nuts. Avoid sugar and salt in all forms because they upset hormonal balance and disturb metabolism, which may cause premature skin aging.

Use power foods within and outside your body. They help rejuvenate your skin, your body envelope, the barometer to good health and long-lasting youth.

See ITCHING.

SMOKING
Power foods that help you kick the habit

Better health and longer life are rewards for kicking the smoking habit. Once you are rid of smoking, you'll improve the physical quality of your daily life and build better resistance to life-shortening ailments such as cancer, heart trouble, emphysema and many other problems.

If you are a regular cigarette smoker, your risk of dying from lung cancer is ten times greater than that of the non-smoker. People aged 25 who have never smoked regularly can expect at least seven years more of power-packed life than those who smoke just one or more packs a day. Twice as many people who are heavy smokers (two packs a day) will die between ages 25 and 65 as those who have never smoked regularly. In the age bracket 40 to 59, strokes kill nearly twice as many smokers as non-smokers. Smokers between 45 and 64 miss 40 percent more working days than do non-smokers.

Smoking Destroys Protection. Tobacco smoke paralyzes the cilia, tiny hairs lining the bronchial tubes, that sweep irritating particles out of the lungs. Without this protection, healthy lung tissue can be injured or even destroyed by these smoke particles.

The basic foundation of health and life calls for internal and external cleanliness and freedom from abuse by tobacco. To help you kick the habit, power foods will build your resistance so that you will be able to put away your cigarettes—forever—in a few days or so.

THE POWER FRUIT THAT ENDED THE SMOKING HABIT IN ONE DAY

Bill D.B. used to smoke like a chimney. Evenings, he smoked with his food, his coffee, his beer. One night he decided to kick the habit after everyone told him he was setting a bad example for his family as well as for youngsters on the school bus he drove daily. Bill D.B. tossed away his package of cigarettes, saying he was finished. Instead of reaching for a cigarette, he reached for a power fruit—*raisins*. Whenever Bill D.B. had the urge to smoke, he reached for a raisin. He would nibble on it, chew and swallow. Often, he would take more than just one raisin. But in one day, this power fruit, simple sun-dried raisins (from supermarket or health store), helped him kick the habit.[1]

[1]"*If You Want to Give Up Cigarettes,*" American Cancer Society, 1979, New York, New York.

Sun-dried raisins contain fructose, a slowly metabolized fruit sugar that energizes the thought waves and the cerebro-endocrinal responses so that there is greater resistance to the smoking urge. Eating a few raisins helps build a shield against the nicotine habit. In one day, Bill D.B. was so invigorated by this power fruit that he kicked a lifelong habit!

POWER FOODS THAT TAKE THE EDGE OFF THE SMOKING URGE

To re-educate your taste buds so that they do not urge you to smoke, try these power foods:

- *Water.* Wash away that acid-churning desire that increases bitter-tasting tongue fluid flow and intensifies the urge to smoke. Drink lots of water daily. Instead of a smoke, reach for a glass of water!
- *Chewy Power Foods.* Use sugarfree candies, gum, mints (from health store or dietetic sections in supermarkets and pharmacies) to give you something to chew whenever you have the urge to hold a cigarette in your mouth. It can be a habit-kicking replacement.
- *Herb Foods.* Chew bits of fresh *ginger* when you start to reach for a cigarette. *Note:* ginger root is aromatic and penetrating, so take it slowly. Ginger root will give you a "burn" similar to that of a cigarette and this gives you a satisfactory substitute. It also helps you feel clean and refreshed to further ease your urge for a cigarette which may "dirty" your mouth and body. Also try a *clove*. It has a refreshing and antiseptic feeling. It tends to divert your oral tissues and tongue buds from the desire to have a smoke and this eases the urge, too. Just bite and chew on a clove slowly as a cigarette substitute.

THE POWER MINERAL THAT BLOCKS THE URGE TO SMOKE

As a mineral, calcium is powerful in being able to soothe the nerve and muscle response that causes the urge to smoke. Calcium blocks this transmitter-dispatched brain message. It binds together with phosphorus to create a feeling of emotional and physical tranquility. The nervous impulse to light up a cigarette is now blocked. With adequate calcium, you can resist this urge.

Power Mineral Program: Have skim milk available. Whenever you have an uncontrollable, twitching, nervous urge to smoke, pour a glass and drink it slowly. The high concentration of calcium will soothe your frazzled oral-tongue tissues and also soothe your brain cells, and this helps block the compulsion.

THE "NIBBLE" WAY TO FREEDOM FROM SMOKING

Nibble celery, carrots, fruit, lettuce to help give you oral satisfaction and reduce your desire to have a cigarette in your mouth. Carry chopped and diced vegetables (raw) with you in a plastic container. Instead of a smoke, just have some of these vegetables. The more you nibble, and the longer it takes you to chew, the less time (and desire) you will have to smoke.

Try Drinking Flaxseed Tea. Ingredients in this herb appear to dull the smoking urge. Just prepare flaxseed tea as you would any tea, then flavor with some lemon juice and honey. Drink several freshly prepared cups daily to help you kick the smoking habit.

Slippery Elm Bark Tea Can Also Help. Use the powdered bark (from health store or herbal pharmacy) with freshly boiled water and some lemon juice and honey for a cup of tea. Drink a few cups daily. You'll find the edge taken off your smoking urge with this herb tea.

With the use of these power foods and beverages, plan *now* to kick the smoking habit. In just three seconds, a cigarette makes your heart beat faster, shoots your blood pressure up, replaces oxygen in your blood with carbon monoxide, and leaves health-destroying life-stealing chemicals to spread through your body. The danger adds up. There is a cumulative effect that causes internal toxemia to build up over a period of time to eventually destroy your youth. Kick the habit *now* and live better— and longer!

See ASTHMA, BREATHING DIFFICULTIES, COUGHS, EMPHYSEMA, SINUSITIS.

SPINAL COLUMN
Power foods that restore youthful flexibility

Your spine is the backbone of better health. Your spinal column consists of about 30 vertebrae (odd-shaped bones that are piled one on top of the other), separated by disks of cartilage (connective tissue) and forming a series of slightly movable joints.

The vertebrae of your spine require the same nourishment as the rest of your body bones. Without proper care, your spine becomes easy to fracture. There may also be a curvature of the spine, creating a stooped gait that can be quite painful as well as unattractive. If deprived of adequate minerals, your bones may become porous, and osteoporosis or thinning may take place, increasing the risk of fracturing. So-called "brittle bones" develop from a spinal column which has become nutritionally weakened and fragile. Your backbone needs to be strong to give support to the rest of your body.

Every body cell is under the influence of the function of healthy spinal nerves. Even the circulatory system with its vascular pump, the heart, and the miles of tubing that make up the blood vessels, is subservient to the modifying control of the central nervous system that is housed in the spine.

Spinal nerves emerge from between the segments of the spine in specially constructed sheaths and are transmitted all over your body. There is an interconnection and interaction of these spinal nerves.

Whatever causes abnormal irritation to these nerves will affect widespread body function. Because these nerves cross between joints and through muscles, and are also responsible for their function, any nutritional deficiency or other abuse of the musculoskeletal system can cause aberrations in the unity of your body. With a disturbance of this balanced interrelation of body systems, age-causing ailments are likely to develop.

Nourish your backbone as a foundation for better health and longer life.

THE POWER FOOD FOR SPINAL STRENGTH

Agatha DelB. felt sharp pains in her spine. When she stooped over to remove an object from a low shelf, she felt agonizing spasms. Trying to straighten up, her spine reacted with recurring knife-like aches that made her cry out with pain. Agatha DelB. began to look exhausted. She walked in a bent-over position that made her look and feel much older than she was. She took her problem to her osteopath who recommended that she fortify her spinal column with a simple, everyday power food that was a highly concentrated source of a bone-nourishing mineral—*yogurt.* Each day, Agatha DelB. had three to four cups of plain or fruit-flavored yogurt. Within seven days, her spinal column felt stronger. Now she was much more flexible. She could touch her fingers to her toes without bending her back and then straighten up again with youthful agility. Agatha DelB. felt herself rejuvenated, thanks to her "forever young" spinal column—and double thanks to yogurt, the powerful mineral food.

Benefits of Yogurt: As a fermented food, its calcium content is intensified because of this pre-digestive type of "ripening." The yogurt calcium works speedily to nourish the spinal bone matrix to fill the sponge-like openings with strong bone.

In particular, yogurt offers calcium in a naturally *acid* medium. This is most beneficial because calcium by itself is not easily deposited in your bones and spinal column. Acid is needed to metabolize the calcium so that it does not coagulate but becomes dispersed to fuse and strengthen the vertebrae, cartilage and nerves so that your spinal column is rejuvenated. Yogurt calcium is a power mineral that strengthens your spine and restores youthful flexibility within a few days! Eat this power food daily for spinal (and body) health.

POWER FRUITS FOR YOUTHFUL SPINE

Fresh fruits and their juices are powerful sources of Vitamin C and bioflavonoids (components of Vitamin C) that create a reaction that will strengthen your spinal column.

The Vitamin C in these power fruits and juices alerts your adrenal glands (storage depot for this nutrient) to release hormones that are involved in strengthening the spinal column, along with your other bones. A malnourished spinal column sends "messages" for Vitamin C to the adrenal glands where it is stored. When you eat power fruit and drink power fruit juices, you dispatch a supply of this Vitamin C to alert your adrenals to release this needed nutrient for spinal nourishment. It is this supply and demand process that helps restore youthful flexibility, health and strength to your spine, and to your entire body.

Spine-Nourishing Program: Daily, enjoy a platter of fresh fruits. Drink fruit juices regularly, too, for Vitamin C boosting powers. Then send a highly concentrated supply of the spine-building power nutrient, Vitamin C.

MAGNESIUM + VITAMIN D = SPINAL STRENGTH

Troubled with wrenching spinal pains, John N.C. would yell out when he made a sudden twist or tried to turn over in bed at night. Chemical liniments irritated and even burned his skin. Wearing a "corset" made him feel like an invalid. John N.C. needed help and he needed it fast. Examined by his company's osteopathic physician, he was told that his spinal column needed nourishment in order to become stronger and more resilient. The physician suggested he try a simple *Spine-Strengthening Potion.* Each day for three days, John N.C. took two glasses of this potion. At the end of the third day, his spine felt strong and no longer ached. He tossed away the liniments and "corset" and now walked, sat, ran, worked and exercised with the spinal agility of a youngster.

What Spine-Strengthening Potion Can Do to Help You. To a glass of fruit juice, add two tablespoons of dolomite powder (from health store or pharmacy) and two tablespoons of cod liver oil. Stir vigorously or blenderize. Now drink one glass in the morning, another freshly prepared glass at noontime, a third one in the evening.

Benefits: The high magnesium content of the dolomite combines with the Vitamin D of the oil and becomes energized by the juice's Vitamin C. In this combination, the nutrients become converted by the liver and kidneys to nourish and invigorate the delicate components of the spinal column, and your general bone structure. *Unique Benefit:* This potion alerts your parathyroid hormone to stimulate bone mineralization. Your parathyroids are situated in the thyroid gland in the front of your neck. This action is brought about by the *combined* efforts of these nutrients in the *Spine-Strengthening Potion.* It works in minutes!

Rebuild and rejuvenate your body through a strong spinal column with the help of power foods and beverages.

See Arthritis, Backaches, Bone Ailments.

STIFFNESS
Power foods that loosen up total body muscles

Muscle is the most abundant tissue in your body. It accounts for some two-fifths of your body weight. Every movement you make, from blinking an eyelash to pushing an object, will call muscles into action to serve your needs. They remain alert and ready to move at the slightest mental or physical command.

"Tight" muscles are traced to inactivity, lack of sufficient use, cell-tissue starvation or deficiency, as well as to blockage that prevents nerve impulses from being transmitted to the muscle fibers. A muscle consists of fibers which are supported and bound together by ordinary connective tissue and are well supplied with blood vessels and nerves. These segments require power food nourishment in order to create youthful muscular flexibility. Without proper nourishment, the segments tend to become tight and there is a sense of "gnarled" muscles that makes you feel stiff all over.

Malnourished muscles react in two ways. They may develop *arthralgia*, meaning pain without inflammation in the joints. Or, they may develop *myalgia*, meaning pain in the muscle fibers. To correct, start with helpful-healing-revitalizing power foods.

THE POWER VITAMIN THAT UNLOCKS YOUR TWISTED MUSCLES

Eleanor Z.K. was troubled with a stubborn "crick in the back" that made her wince whenever she tried to do simple household chores, reach for a package on a high supermarket shelf or even water her backyard garden. Her muscles felt knotted up and painfully tight. Sometimes she would cry out, with tears running down her face, when a tight wincing pain seized her in a vise-like grip. Eleanor Z.K. asked her nurse-neighbor for some help and was told that she needed to boost her intake of B-complex vitamins. She did this with a simple power food—*brewer's yeast.* She would sprinkle it over salads, use it in soups, stews, casseroles, blenderize it with fruit and vegetable juices. Within five days, her muscles were "unlocked" and the twisted feeling had slackened. Soon, Eleanor Z.K. could do her housework, reach in all directions without any muscle pain. She uses brewer's yeast daily to keep her muscles young—along with the rest of her body.

Power Vitamin Benefit: The Vitamin B-complex group is highly potent and concentrated in brewer's yeast, available in health stores and pharmacies. This vitamin family works together to nourish the cell-tissue components of muscle fiber and to dissolve the blockage so that nerve impulses are now able to freely transmit messages. This is the key to "unlocking" tight muscles. The power vitamin group also creates relaxation of *arthralgia*, cools any feeling of inflammation, and soothes muscle fibers to ease *myalgia.* Through more vigorously healthy message conduction in the muscle network, without blockage, the B-complex vitamins of brewer's yeast can help ease stress and strain and promote more youthful agility of the total body muscles.

Two Power Fruits for Flexible Muscles. The orange and the banana are power fruits because they contain high amounts of potassium. This mineral works with sodium in the extracellular fluid of cell-muscle tissues to regulate blood pH (acid-alkaline balance) nerve conduction and muscle contraction. A deficiency of potassium will cause these muscle tissues to tighten up and constrict, thereby bringing on the painful spasms that cause so much distress. To potassium-nourish your muscles, just eat several bananas daily; drink several glasses of orange juice and eat oranges, too, each day. You'll be boosting muscle and body health through potassium power.

Muscle-Soothing Home Remedies. Warm baths, stretching exercises, bed rest are important to help relax distressed muscles. If you work on hard floors, wear sponge-soled shoes for better comfort. If you are a desk worker, correct chair height to prevent muscle strain. Increase your daily walking, bicycling, jogging and general exercises. Keep your muscles more active so they do not atrophy. Even with power nourishment, your muscles may not be loosened up if you remain sluggish or inactive. Raspberry herb tea is said to be muscle-nourishing and soothing. Yogurt and dairy products offer important calcium which helps nerve-muscle contraction, so eat these power foods daily. Muscles also require *nitrogen* for strength and vigor. Feed this principal air component to your muscles through protein from a vegetable or animal source. This includes lean meat, fish, dairy products, seeds, beans, nuts and whole grains. Eat these foods daily for muscle-nourishing *nitrogen* so you'll be able to move with the agility of a youngster.

Alert yourself to meet the responsibilities of a happiness-filled lifestyle. Loosen up total body muscles, erase stiffness and enjoy productive years of abundant and youthful health.

See Arteriosclerosis, Arthritis, Backache, Bursitis, Leg and Foot Problems, Muscular Aches, Spinal Column.

"SWEET TOOTH" Power foods that help conquer this habit

The desire for sugar can be controlled by easing the emotional drive responsible for this "sweet tooth" compulsion. To better motivate yourself to use power foods to help conquer the "sugarholic" habit, you should know the health risks caused by eating or drinking sweets.

Sugar in any form has a cariogenic (decay-causing) effect on the teeth. This sweet will also build up calories and add weight that will be difficult to melt away. Sugar is believed to boost the levels of triglycerides in the bloodstream, increase cholesterol deposits and thereby enhance the risk of hypertension as well as arteriosclerosis and heart trouble. Your metabolism may react harshly to an overload of sugar and this may cause cell-tissue destruction and symptoms of ill health and premature aging. Sugar also upsets gland-hormone balance and is involved in the malfunctioning of the pancreas. This disrupts a normal release of insulin and problems of diabetes result. Sugar will cause an up-and-down tug of war with your blood sugar levels to induce hypoglycemia and related emotional-physical disturbances. Sugar is considered a mischief-maker in your system. Do not take this dissident into your body and you will enjoy better health and extra years of youthful life.

THE POWER TONIC THAT CONTROLS YOUR "SWEET TOOTH"

Herbert J.R. was able to control his "sweet tooth" and conquer the habit to eat sweets by beginning each meal with a simple, tasty and effective power tonic.

In a glass of fruit juice, stir one tablespoon of brewer's yeast powder. Stir vigorously or blenderize. Then sip slowly.

Benefits: The brewer's yeast is a highly concentrated source of an active mineral, chromium, which influences the glucose tolerance factor that is involved with the hypothalamus-initiated urge to have something sweet. The fructose of the fruit juice is used by the chromium to offer you a steady satisfaction of the appetite for sweets, and this helps to control and conquer the urge to eat sugar or sugar-containing foods. This power tonic is especially effective at the *start* of a meal when your appetite is big and you have the strongest urge to gobble down sweets. This urge is controlled through the chromium-fructose combination in this power tonic. Plan to drink a freshly prepared glass of this tonic before each meal. You will be able to block the sugar urge almost immediately and kick the habit within a day or less!

POWER FOOD SNACKS THAT HELP YOU CONQUER THE SWEET-NIBBLING HABIT

Whenever you have the urge for something sweet, nibble on these power food snacks as a soothing and satisfying substitute: seeds, nuts, hard-boiled eggs, any raw vegetable that is chewy such as celery, carrots, lettuce, even cabbage. Carry a plastic bag of freshly cut or diced raw vegetables and snack whenever you want to sweet-nibble. Have salt-free, sugar-free popcorn, soda crackers, whole grain toast, hard rolls. The white sugar habit can be replaced by a *natural* sugar habit in the form of fruits such as oranges, grapefruit, tangerines, apricots, plums, apples, pears, peaches, nectarines, cherries, strawberries, grapes, melons, avocados, pineapples. Just snack and nibble on these foods whenever you have a compulsion to eat something sweet. You'll feel satisfied in a matter of minutes and be free of the urge to nibble on white sugar items.

HOW TO RINSE AWAY YOUR "SWEET TOOTH"

The so-called "sweet tooth" is actually a sugar urge that is often prompted by a salivary increase in the taste buds on the tongue. Known as papillae (small, rounded elevations), they become aroused, stimulated by your hypothalamus, to release saliva which tends to give you an urge to have something sweet. To tame this urge, try a simple mouth and tongue rinse: in a glass of warm water, put one teaspoon of ordinary baking soda. Dissolve. Then rinse out your mouth. The minerals in the baking soda tend to take the "bite" off the edge of your tongue and soothe the papillae so your "sweet tooth" urge is actually rinsed away. Whenever you feel this tongue-burning sensation, nip the "sweet tooth" in the bud with this simple mouth and tongue rinse. It works within minutes!

With the use of these power tonics, snacks and rinse, you should be able to control and conquer your "sweet tooth" habit in a short while. You'll feel much healthier for it, too.

See Diabetes, Digestive Disturbances, Fatigue, Low Blood Sugar, Mouth Disorders, Weight Control.

TREMBLING
Power foods that soothe shakes and flutters

Whether called the "shakes" or delirium tremens or uncontrollable trembling, this constant nervous shudder is a drain on your health resources. Excessive shakes and flutters will cause an intensification of your metabolism and this causes an upset of your normal body rhythm. Such an imbalance will disrupt the delicate rhythm of your body glands and thus cause uneven hormone release so that you reduce your body's defenses against illness.

If trembling is unrelieved, it may lead to related problems such as nervous tics or muscular tightness which results in slow and jerky movements. Routine actions such as rising from a chair become difficult. The trembling person tends to experience cramp-like pains in the arm and legs, even when at rest. This may lead to such debilitation that the temptation is to just lie in bed, almost like an invalid. If the shakes persist and are not relieved, the risk of becoming permanently bed-bound is very strong.

Repeated trembling is a drain on the body's energy reserves and needs to be corrected with the use of high-vitamin power foods. In particular, power foods that are prime sources of the B-complex vitamins can correct the basic cause of most shakes and restore soothing comfort to the entire body.

THE GRAIN THAT SOOTHES NERVOUS TREMBLES AND SHAKES

Arlene O'C. developed a nervous trembling type of tic that made her shake her arms, shoulders, even her legs, for moments or sometimes an hour—or even overnight. Arlene O'C. could not hold a cup in her hand because the trembling caused it to fall and break! She was examined by an orthomolecular neurologist (nerve specialist who uses nutritional therapy where advisable) who said that this purposeless repetitive movement of a muscle was caused by a deficiency of an important B-complex vitamin—choline. He told her to take this vitamin in supplement form and also to boost intake through a few foods. Within four days, the trembling ended. Her hands were as steady as a youngster's. She looked radiantly healthy. Thanks to a special grain food, she had healed the problem that plagued her for months.

Power Grain Food: Brewer's yeast is this power grain food. It is a highly concentrated source of choline. This particular B-complex vitamin is needed to control the involuntary trembling and shaking that is so distressful.

Benefit: Trembling is usually caused if there is a metabolic imbalance of two brain substances: dopamine and acetylcholine. These two substances need to send messages between nerve cells which are then "commanded" to control muscle function throughout the body. If there is a healthy balance of both dopamine and acetylcholine, nerve impulses may be healthfully passed along. But if there is a decrease of either dopamine or acetylcholine (or both), then the delicate balance is upset. Nerve signals tend to become confused. This leads to trembling and uncontrollable shakes. Adding *choline* through a power food such as brewer's yeast helps make up the deficiency, restores better balance, and gives the brain a sufficient amount of dopamine and acetylcholine to transmit muscle-controlling messages. With the use of this power grain, brewer's yeast, the muscle-controlling messages are even and tranquil. Trembling is eliminated.

Suggestion: Use brewer's yeast, a potent brain-feeding source of choline, as part of your daily cereal, in soups, stews, casseroles, baked dishes of all sorts. Add to a fruit or vegetable juice and drink as a Shake-Stopping Potion at least once or twice a day. The high choline content will speedily control trembling and the shakes will calm down. So will the rest of your body.

Power Mineral for Ending of Shakes and Flutters. Magnesium is a power mineral that will help to diminish and then end the uncontrollable shakes and flutters that create worsening symptoms if unchecked. Magnesium mobilizes calcium from the bones and uses it to soothe frazzled nerves. Magnesium and calcium are also used to strengthen the brain so it can release healthy balances of the important dopamine and acetylcholine substances that can end shakes and flutters. Magnesium is available in supplements. Another good source is any green, leafy vegetable, especially as part of the chlorophyl molecule. Eat this type of vegetable raw, as part of a salad. Seafoods also contain ample amounts of shake-ending magnesium.

Restore brain wave balance to your body with the help of power foods and you'll enjoy freedom from trembling, shakes and flutters.

See Alcoholism, Dizziness, Fatigue, Itching, Muscular Aches, Nervousness.

ULCERS
Power foods that promote relief and healing

An ulcer is a condition in which there is the erosion or destruction of skin or mucous membrane of the lining of the stomach. A *peptic* ulcer affects the inner lining. A *gastric* ulcer affects the digestive section of the lining. Symptoms may range from burning to an agonizing reaction when ordinary, everyday foods and drinks are consumed. There are times when the ulcer is not felt so you are lulled into an illusion of healing. But the ulcer remains dormant, acting up later on when the digestive system is irritated to the slightest degree.

Basic Problem: In a healthy digestive system, your stomach lining is strong enough so that when strong acids and juices are released to metabolize food, there is no irritation. But in an ulcer condition, this basic defense of the stomach's lining against digestive acids has weakened. Any irritation of this opening will cause the burning sensation. Continued irritation of this sensitive region will give rise to a sore or a wound, and this is known as the ulcer.

Caution: If an ulcer is not healed or treated, the risk is high that it will "perforate." It tends to erode through the wall of the stomach. This allows the stomach's contents to spill over into the abdominal region. If this happens, there is a serious consequence of vomiting blood. There may be accompanying internal bleeding as well as blood in the stool. This indicates immediate need for corrective measures.

Basic Ulcer Healing Suggestions: Shield yourself from any emotional or physical upset. It triggers an outpouring of stomach acid (even if you've not eaten anything for hours) and this will cause ulcer flare-up and burning. Eliminate coffee and tea because their caffeine-tannic acid content irritates your delicate and inflamed stomach tissues and causes burning reactions. Eliminate tobacco and alcohol because of their erosion-causing qualities. Medications may also be irritating, so be sure to follow your doctor's suggestions. Aspirin tends to create further erosion and should generally be eliminated.

Small Meals Are Ulcer-Soothing. Adjust your eating program. Divide your meals into smaller portions. Large amounts of food are taxing to your irritated stomach and will cause an excessive outpouring of acid that is inflamed and hurtful. Smaller meals will reduce acid flow to a level your digestive tract can accommodate with minimal discomfort. Foods should be neither too hot nor too cold. Fried foods should be avoided because their fat content is irritating and brings on a flow of burning acid.

SOOTHE AND HEAL STOMACH ULCERS WITH POWER OIL

Wheat germ oil is a powerful source of Vitamin E, an emollient that coats the lining of the stomach and acts as a mucilaginous shield against corrosive acids. Plan to use wheat germ oil as part of a salad dressing or combined in vegetable juices, at least twice daily.

Suggestion: Before you begin any meal, take four tablespoons of wheat germ oil. *Benefit:* The coating action of the Vitamin E in the oil has a significant prophylactic benefit and facilitates the healing process. It coats the open sore and shields against burning from stomach acid.

HEAL ULCERS WITH POWER VITAMIN

Vitamin A has the unique ability to cause the stomach membranes to secrete a continuous mucus which then covers the cells and tissues and protects them from stomach acids which might otherwise irritate and inflame. Vitamin A causes this mucus-releasing response and this promotes swifter healing of ulcers which are now free from irritation.

Vitamin A is able to stimulate the epithelial cells (those which line tissues of the stomach) to reproduce at a healthier rate to replace those that have been burned out. This causes increased mucus and therefore greater protection at the same time. In many ulcer situations, there is a corresponding deficiency of Vitamin A.

Power Vitamin Sources: Rich-colored fresh fruits and vegetables, dairy products, eggs, margarine, fish liver oils, desiccated liver. *Suggestion:* Start off each meal with a fresh raw fruit or vegetable salad sprinkled with desiccated liver and flavored with three tablespoons of wheat germ oil. This boosts Vitamin A and also Vitamin E protection and accelerates healing.

Ulcer-Healing Power Tonic: To a glass of fresh fruit or vegetable juice, add two tablespoons of wheat germ oil and two tablespoons of any fish liver oil (available as mint flavored, if preferred). Stir or blenderize. Sip slowly.

Benefit: You have a powerhouse of Vitamins A and E together with fructose to enhance their effectiveness in speedily healing your digestive tract. In a matter of moments, there is an increase in protective mucus and also the creation of new epithelial cells needed to hasten the healing of the open sore. Drink several glasses of this *Ulcer-Healing Power Tonic* for fast and effective relief.

Power Foods for Basic Ulcer Healing

- *Cucumber Juice.* A prime source of important trace elements that cool inflammation and hasten healing.
- *Avocado Fast.* For two days, eat nothing but sliced avocados. The polyunsaturated fatty acids and oils are especially soothing and pampering to open sores and hasten healing.
- *Carrot Juice.* A good source of carotene, which is transformed into Vitamin A to rebuild the destroyed cells of the stomach lining.
- *Papaya.* Eat this fruit regularly; it contains enzymes which improve the digestive power of your stomach and help replenish the stomach lining.
- *Barley.* Freshly prepared barley with a bit of honey for flavoring is a good source of the B-complex vitamins which are needed to soothe digestive unrest and promote swifter healing of open sores. These vitamins act as emollients on the irritated wounds.
- *Herb Healer.* Take a half-teaspoon of powdered cloves or oil of cloves (from health store or herbal pharmacy) and hold in your mouth until dissolved. It should be mixed well with

saliva. Repeat several times daily. Oils in this herb help to coat the digestive tract and cool burning in a matter of minutes.

You can eat and drink your way (with power foods) to relief and healing of ulcers.

See Digestive Disturbances.

URINARY PROBLEMS Power foods that help establish normal flow

Difficulty in emptying the bladder, whether occasional or frequent, is a symptom of infection or blocking of the organs of urination. These include the kidneys, bladder, prostate (in males), pancreas. If there is scanty urine or excessive (night) urination, discomfort or discoloration, corrective healing measures should be taken to help establish a normal flow.

Urinary problems are often traced to environmental or metabolic conditions. There may be inflammation without bacteria in the urine: or the situation can be reversed so that there is bacteria in the urine but no signs of inflammation or infection. To help correct the cause, the use of improved living methods along with power foods can ease distress and reestablish normal release of wastes.

THE POWER VITAMIN THAT HELPS MALE URINE DIFFICULTIES

Sidney I.Y. was troubled with bouts of excessive urination, sometimes having to get up at night to empty his bladder. Sometimes he suffered from incontinence (the inability to restrain the discharge of urine from the body). At still other times he had difficulty as he strained to urinate. Worried, he asked his urologist for help. After his condition was diagnosed, he was told to boost his intake of a power vitamin. Sidney I.Y. increased his daily dose of this vitamin, and in seven days his urine problems were solved and he had established a normal flow.

Power Vitamin: Everyday Vitamin C, found in citrus fruits and their juice, is able to control any rish of urinary infection and also correct blockage causes of bladder irregularities.

Benefits: Vitamin C in fruit juice helps to soothe inflammation and irritations by washing out phosphatic crystals, grain-like substances that tend to block the ducts through which urine passes. Vitamin C has the catalytic power to saturate these phosphatic crystals, create a needed acid environment, then force these same phosphatic crystals into a liquefied condition. As a liquid, they can be washed out of the system. This power vitamin is able to acidify the crystals and the urine and cleanse the urethral canal and related ducts.

Suggestion: Drink citrus fruit juices regularly. Eat the fruits, too. Vitamin C food supplements are available. Cranberry juice is another concentrated source of this power vitamin. It increases needed acidification to break down accumulated phosphatic crystals, free the channels of blockage and restore normal flow.

THE POWER BEVERAGE THAT CORRECTS INCONTINENCE

May K.V. had difficulties in controlling urination. Medications gave her diarrhea and other side effects. She had to find a natural way to heal her condition. A herbal pharmacist suggested a folk remedy. She tried it, and within two days she could control her urination. Incontinence was ended. She felt wonderful. She now enjoys an established normal flow as a result of drinking one cup of this power beverage each day.

Power Beverage: Use bean pods! (Not canned, dried or frozen.) Buy fresh stringbeans, shell them, then use the pods. Boil a half-cup of washed and cut-up bean pods in two quarts of water. Strain carefully. Let cool. If necessary, strain again. Drink one glass every two hours. Properties in the bean pods appear to be "liberated" by the boiling, and help to correct urinary retention and to wash out gravel blockage.

Less Sugar = Better Bladder Health. The kidney-bladder network may react to the high metabolic rate of processed sugar.

This may cause organ-allergy. A reaction may be that of excessive urination. The central nervous system becomes upset by the intake of sugar and causes a variety of unpleasant symptoms such as kidney-bladder distress. Since sugar filters through these organs, the irritation may lead to urine distress. If you consume less sugar (better yet, none at all!), you'll help establish better metabolic balance and a soothed kidney-bladder combo. You'll be able to experience natural elimination with no excesses in either extreme.

Powdered Vervain Tea. This herbal tea (health stores and pharmacies) is believed to contain ingredients that will help remove bladder obstructions and stimulate normal flow of urine. Drink it daily.

Herb Healers. The use of caraway, sweet fennel, anise will help increase elimination of wastes. Use for tea, or add to soups, stews, casseroles, breads. Tasty and healing at the same time. Use singly or in combination.

Basic Suggestions: Do not "shock" your system with very hot or very cold foods or beverages. Avoid excessively spiced foods. Eat slowly. Take frequent comfortably warm baths. Eliminate "hot" seasoned foods which upset your kidney-bladder organs. Clothing should not be so tight as to constrict these and related organs. Keep your feet warm. This avoids chilling which upsets normal flow.

With the use of power foods and beverages and basic health suggestions, you should be able to help establish normal flow of urine and enjoy a cleansed system.

See Bladder, Colitis, Constipation, Cramps, Diarrhea, Kidneys, Prostate, Sex-Related Disorders, Sexual Power.

VARICOSE VEINS
Power foods that smooth away leg ulcers

Varicose veins develop when valves in the veins have become weakened, or when walls of the veins are weak. In time, they may give way under pressure of blood and sag outward at the site of the valves. As a result, the valves cannot close tightly to regulate the flow of blood. This, in turn, further increases the pressure of blood against the vein walls.

The trouble may start high in the deep veins and extend to the communicating and surface veins. As the pressure increases, valve after valve along the veins may be affected. Veins in the legs must support a heavy column of blood as it flows back to the heart. When the pressure in the veins is above normal levels, some of the veins in the legs balloon out and become varicosed.

Basic Causes: There may be factors of heredity. Basically, any extra strain on the circulation of blood in the veins can affect the valves. Standing still for a long time places great strain on the veins. Sitting for long hours is almost as bad. Whatever interferes with circulation of the blood in the veins, including tight clothing such as girdles or garters, can cause varicose veins to become worse. If a vein is injured and phlebitis (inflammation) develops, the valves may be involved. Valves can also be affected by excessive overweight. Some elderly people develop this problem because the veins tend to lose their elasticity with aging. The muscles supporting them weaken and varicosities occur.

POWER VITAMIN THAT OPENS UP CLOGGED VEINS

Vitamin E, taken as a supplement or in wheat germ oil or whole grains such as wheat germ and brain, appears to have a power effect in helping to open up clogged veins.

Power Benefit: This power vitamin produces collateral circulation around the obstructed deep veins by calling into play the unused networks of veins lying in wait for emergency utilizations. Vitamin E has the unique power of enabling tissues to utilize oxygen better. This helps to open up and heal the devitalized and congested tissues. The clogging is done away with because of the fibrinolytic (fibrin-dissolving) power of Vitamin E.

Suggestion: Whether in the form of a supplement or oil or grain, take Vitamin E daily. Your entire body and your veins will respond with better health through free-flowing blood.

Okra: Vein Cleanser. The vegetable, okra, is a prime source of both silicon and selenium, two minerals that help open clogged veins, and then strengthen capillaries. They push blood out of congested sites and this eases the distress of varicose veins.

Circulation-Boosting Tips for Healthier Veins

Begin by avoiding prolonged standing or sitting because this chokes off circulation; blood then accumulates in your lower legs and around your ankles and your veins are distended. Follow these circulation-boosting tips:

1. When on a long plane or train trip, get up and walk around every half hour. Or on a long auto trip, stop once in a while. Get out to stretch your legs.
2. When reading, try to keep your feet elevated. Rest your legs on a chair, stool or hassock. The executive who sits with his feet on the desk has the right idea!
3. Exercise improves your circulation. Walking is beneficial. The movements of leg muscles help push the blood upward. Swimming or walking in deep water does much the same thing; the great pressure of the water against your legs helps move blood up the veins.
4. Sleeping with your feet raised slightly above the level of your heart helps the blood flow away from your ankles.
5. If possible, raise the foot of your bed by placing six-inch-high blocks under the bedposts at the foot end. This gives better support than simply raising the mattress.
6. Round garters should never be worn. They cut off the venous circulation, thus raising pressure in the veins and increasing the risk of varicosities. Avoid any constriction.
7. Elastic girdles should not be worn continuously—especially when you will be seated for a long time, such as at a desk, or during any plane, train, bus or auto trip. They bunch up and hamper the return flow of blood. This increases the pressure of the blood in the veins and gives rise to varicose veins.

Improve your leg (and body) circulation with the use of power foods and the health tips listed above. You will help to smooth away leg ulcers for better health and a more youthfully attractive body.

See Foot Problems, Hemorrhoids, Leg and Foot Problems.

WEAKNESS
Power foods that revitalize your body from head to toe

Weakness, tiredness, fatigue—no matter what you call it, it makes you look and feel much older than your years. An occasional feeling of weakness is no cause for alarm. It means you need to rest. But if you feel weak when you awaken in the morning, if you feel tired when standing on line for just a few moments, if you experience fatigue after doing ordinary home or business chores for a little while, then your body's capacity for youthful energy needs to be revitalized.

Weakness or fatigue is usually caused when there is a lowering of body defenses against the toxins that induce this feeling of tiredness that appears to persist and even worsen as the hours and days go on. Weakness is usually a symptom of inadequate nutrition in the glandular network as well as in the bloodstream. There may be accompanying symptoms such as headaches, fever, shortness of breath, muscular aches as well as rapid heartbeat. These all signify a need for corrective nutrition, improved living methods and the use of power foods for total revitalization.

HOW TO WAKE UP YOUR SLEEPING THYROID GLAND

To revitalize your body from head to toe, use power foods to wake up your sleeping thyroid gland. This organ may become sluggish, and this will cause that "always tired" feeling that is making you look and feel much older than you are.

Location, Function, Energy Source. Situated in the front of your neck, this energy-boosting gland consists of two lobes, one on either side of the Adam's apple. The thyroid produces a hormone, *thyroxine*, which consists of iodine plus the amino acid tyrosine. These nutrients are used to accelerate the release of energy in your tissues via the combustion of glucose. When this happens, breathing and blood circulation are increased to give you more oxygen. Your body and your mind feel revitalized. Your muscles and related body organs are now stimulated. You no longer feel weak but have a sensation of exhilaration and revitalization from head to toe.

All of this youthful vitality is possible through a well-nourished thyroid gland. Its nutrient-carrying hormone can create this chain reaction of youthful stimulation in a matter of moments!

Power Food That Energizes Thyroxine Release. Seafood is a prime source of iodine, the mineral that stimulates the thyroid, then becomes part of the hormone together with available tyrosine to trigger a set of healthy and revitalized processes throughout your body to make you look and feel alert and responsive to activities in your midst. *Suggestion:* Plan to eat seafood as often as possible. It's an energy-producing power food.

The Seasoning That Puts Spice in Your Life. Feel weak? Lethargic? "Don't care any more" type of attitude? Then it's time you woke up your tired thyroid and took part in the exciting world in your midst. Do this with a seasoning that is sure to put spice into your life. It's *kelp*. This is a powder made from seaweed grown in the iodine-rich beds of the deep ocean. Available in health stores and many supermarkets, it contains potassium and magnesium which work with iodine to wake up your tired thyroid and open a new threshold to energy-filled living. Just use kelp as a tangy substitute for table salt in cooking as well as at the table. Within moments after kelp enters your digestive system, its iodine content is released and sent to your thyroid gland where it initiates a powerful thyroxine release to give you a feeling of total revitalization from head to toe. It can work almost at once! (Kelp tablets are available at health stores and pharmacies.)

Be Energetic with B-Complex Vitamins. Found in whole grains such as wheat germ, rice polishings, brewer's yeast (which has at least 10 of these B-complex vitamins together with 16 protein factors including tyrosine which joins with iodine to energize thyroxine release) and desiccated liver. Use these whole grain foods daily. You'll erase weakness and develop new physical strength from head to toe with their energizing vitamins.

Kelp + Brewer's Yeast + Fruit Juice = Youthful Energy. To a glass of citrus fruit juice, add one-half teaspoon of kelp and one tablespoon of brewer's yeast. Blenderize. Drink slowly.

Benefit: The Vitamin C energized enzymes of the fruit juice seize hold of the kelp iodine and the yeast tyrosine to supercharge your thyroid to produce youthful energy in a matter of moments. Just one glass of this power food energy tonic and you'll enjoy day-long vigor and stamina!

With the help of everyday tasty, tangy and tart power foods, you can help revitalize your body from head to toe—in minutes.

WEIGHT CONTROL
Power foods that help keep you slim and trim

With the use of power foods, you can shape up—and keep in shape. Weight control is possible when you follow some basic rules about eating and learn how to cut down on excessive calorie build-up. Here are some starter suggestions:

1. Use a smaller dinner plate. It looks more satisfying than a large, empty looking plate.
2. Eat slowly and you will be satisfied with less.
3. Raw vegetables are great weight-controlling power foods. Try carrot sticks, cucumber sticks, radishes, celery sticks. Try fresh grapefruit. Its sections are wonderfully juicy and refreshing. *Benefit:* The grapefruit is much lower in calories than sweets and will give you a longer-lasting energy boost because of its natural fructose and Vitamin C. *Tip:* Have a bowl of sections handy in your refrigerator. Nibble a few

sections between meals to reduce the temptation to eat high-calorie snacks.

4. Try drinking a glass of citrus fruit juice with your meal. It helps you feel more satisfied with less food.
5. Burn up unwanted calories with healthful exercises such as walking, bicycling, swimming, jogging.

How to Use Chart: Note the high calorie foods. Plan to restrict or eliminate them. If you must take them, plan to burn up their calories through any of the four suggested exercises. Now look at the low calorie foods. These are your *power* foods because they give you good nutrition with fewer calories. Plan to eat more of these.

See Digestive Disturbances, "Sweet Tooth."

Suggestions: Cut back on hard fats as much as possible. Switch to more fish and poultry with fat trimmed off. Eliminate refined sugar from cooking, from the shaker and from processed foods. Read labels. Cook lean. Eat lean. Substitute herbs, apple cider vinegar, spices, lemon juice for flavorings. These satisfy without adding calories as do water-absorbing table salt, sugar, ketchup, mustard and other harsh seasonings.

Power Food Fat-Melting Beverage. In a glass of grapefruit juice, stir one tablespoon of apple cider vinegar and two tablespoons of honey. Blenderize for better assimilation. Drink a half hour before a meal.

Benefit: This fat-melting beverage gives you a powerhouse of potassium from the apple cider vinegar which is energized by the fruit juice and combined with the vigor of the honey minerals to regulate your thyroid and help control your appetite. The potassium is an effective hormone stimulant that can promote better fat melting that helps control your weight.

Enjoy your power foods, follow the simple guidelines for control of weight, plan to burn up added calories through any of the easy exercises and you should be able to keep slim and trim and youthful, too.

See Circulation, Fainting, Fatigue, Low Blood Sugar, Trembling.

Calorie Counter and Energy Equivalents

Number of minutes of exercise required to expend the caloric energy of the food items shown below

		Food Energy - Calories	1) Walking (min)	2) Bicycling (min)	3) Swimming (min)	4) Jogging (min)
Beverages Alcoholic	Beer (12 fl oz)	150	29	23	18	15
	Gin (1-1/2 fl oz)	105	20	16	12	10
	Rye Whisky (1-1/2 fl oz)	105	20	16	12	10
	Vodka (1-1/2 fl. oz)	105	20	16	12	10
	Wine, dessert (6 fl oz)	233	45	36	27	23
	table (6 fl oz)	145	28	22	17	14
Beverages, Non-alcoholic	Coffee cream & sugar (2 cups)	86	17	13	10	9
	Cream (1 tbsp)	30	6	5	4	3
	Fruit drinks (1 cup)	135	26	21	16	14
	Milk, Whole 3.5% fat (1 cup)	160	31	25	19	16
	Non fat skim (1 cup)	90	17	14	11	9
	Partially skimmed 2% fat 1 cup)	123	24	19	14	12
	Milkshake (1 cup)	280	54	43	33	28
	Soft drinks cola 10 fl oz)	121	23	19	14	12
	ginger ale (10 fl oz)	95	18	15	11	10
	Tea with cream & sugar (2 cups)	86	17	13	10	9
Breads & Cereals	Bread Rye 1 slice	73	14	11	9	8
	White enriched 1 slice)	82	16	12	10	8
	Whole wheat 1 slice)	72	14	11	8	7
	Breakfast cereals cooked					
	Cream of wheat (1 cup)	105	20	16	12	10
	Oatmeal (1 cup)	130	25	20	15	13
	Breakfast cereals, dry ready-to-eat					
	Bran flakes (3/4 cup)	104	20	16	12	10
	Cornflakes (1 cup)	80	15	12	9	8
	Puffed oats, presweetened (3 4 cup)	107	21	16	13	11
	Puffed rice, presweetened (1 cup)	120	23	18	14	12
	Wheat flakes (1 cup)	105	20	16	12	11
	Puffed wheat presweetened (1 cup)	80	15	12	9	8
	Shredded wheat (1 biscuit = 12 spoon size)	80	15	12	9	8
	Macaroni & cheese (1 cup)	430	83	66	51	43
	Noodles (1 2 cup)	100	19	15	12	10
	Pancakes, plain (1 6" dia)	90	17	14	11	9
	with butter & syrup (1. 6" dia)	310	60	48	36	31
	Rolls and buns					
	White dinner roll (1)	90	17	14	11	9
	Hamburg or hot dog bun (1)	164	32	25	19	16
	Whole wheat roll (1)	79	15	12	9	8
	Spaghetti, cooked (1/2 cup)	78	15	12	9	8
	Spaghetti & meat sauce (1 cup)	330	63	51	39	33
	Spaghetti & tomato sauce (1 cup)	145	28	22	17	14
	Waffles, plain (1 6' dia)	180	35	28	21	18
	with butter & syrup (1. 6' dia)	400	77	62	47	40
Desserts	Cakes					
	Devil's Food	235	45	36	28	24
	White, with icing	400	77	62	47	40
	Candy					
	Hard candy (1 oz)	110	21	17	13	11
	Marshmallows (1 oz)	90	17	14	11	9
	Milk chocolate bars, all varieties (1-1/4 oz)	168	32	26	20	17
	Chelsea bun, cinnamon bun (1)	158	30	24	19	16
	Cookies, Brownies with nuts (1)	95	18	15	12	10
	Chocolate chip or fig bars (1)	50	10	8	6	5
	Chocolate marshmallow (1)	75	14	12	9	8
	Social tea or arrowroot (1)	20	4	3	2	2
	Oatmeal, commercial (1)	86	17	13	10	9
	Doughnuts (1)	125	24	19	15	12
	Gelatin desserts (3/4 cup)	60	12	9	7	6
	Ice cream (3/4 cup)	191	37	29	22	19
	Pies, Apple (1 sector)	410	79	63	48	41
	Cherry (1 sector)	387	74	60	46	39
	Custard (1 sector)	327	63	50	38	33
	Lemon meringue (1 sector)	357	69	55	42	36
	Pudding instant (1 2 cup)	182	35	28	21	18
	rice or tapioca 1 2 cup)	141	27	22	17	14

Number of minutes of exercise required to expend the caloric energy of the food items shown below

		Food Energy-Calories	1) Walking (min)	2) Bicycling (min)	3) Swimming (min)	4) Jogging (min)
Fruits & Fruit Juices	Apples raw 1 med 2-1 2" dia.)	87	17	13	10	9
	Apple juice - Vit C Added (1 2 cup)	60	12	9	7	6
	Apple sauce - sweetened (1/2 cup)	115	22	18	14	12
	unsweetened	50	10	8	6	5
	Bananas (1)	100	19	15	12	10
	Blueberries (3/4 cup)	64	12	10	8	6
	Cantaloupe (1 4)	30	6	5	4	3
	Cherries raw (1/2 cup)	59	11	9	7	6
	Grapefruit (1 2 cup)	45	9	7	5	4
	Grapefruit juice (1/2 cup)	48	9	7	6	5
	Grapes (1 2 cup)	32	6	5	4	3
	Nectarines (1 medium)	96	18	15	11	10
	Oranges (1) or orange juice (1/2 cup)	60	12	9	7	6
	Peaches, raw (1)	35	7	5	4	4
	canned (1/2 cup)	100	19	15	12	10
	Pears raw 1) or canned (1 2 cup)	100	19	15	12	10
	Pineapple raw (1 2 cup)	38	7	6	4	4
	canned with syrup (1 2 cup)	98	19	15	12	10
	Plums raw (1)	25	5	4	3	2
	canned (1/2 cup)	102	20	16	12	10
	Raisins (1 oz)	80	15	12	9	8
	Raspberries (3/4 cup)	52	10	8	6	5
	Rhubarb cooked 1 2 cup)	192	37	30	23	19
	Strawberries (3/4 cup)	41	8	6	5	4
	Tangerines (1)	40	8	6	5	4
Meats	Bacon side (3 slices)	135	25	21	16	14
	Canadian or back	245	47	38	29	24
	Beef & vegetable stew (1 cup)	210	40	32	25	21
	Beef cooked					
	Ground beef, broiled, lean (3 oz)	185	36	28	22	18
	Ground beef broiled, regular (3 oz)	245	47	38	29	24
	Rib roast (3 oz)	375	72	58	44	38
	Pot roast (3 oz)	245	47	38	29	24
	Sirloin steak (3 oz)	330	63	51	39	33
	Ham (3 oz)	245	47	38	29	24
	Lamb chop (1 bone in)	400	77	62	47	40
	(1 no bone)	400	77	62	47	40
	Lamb, leg roast (3 oz)*	235	45	36	28	24
	Liver beef calf chicken or pork, fried (2 oz)	130	25	20	15	13
	Lunch meats, canned (1 oz)	83	16	13	10	8
	Pork, chop (1)	260	50	40	31	26
	roast (3 oz)	310	60	48	36	31
	Sausages (3 links)	188	37	29	22	19
	Veal, cutlet (3 oz)	185	36	28	22	19
	roast (3 oz)	230	44	35	27	23
Poultry & Eggs	Chicken					
	Breast, fried (1/2 breast = 3.3 oz) with bone	155	29	24	18	16
	Meat only (.5625 cup diced = 3 oz)	115	22	18	14	12
	Eggs					
	Boiled or poached (1)	80	15	12	9	8
	Scrambled or fried (1)	110	21	17	13	11
Sandwiches & Snacks	Crackers					
	Graham 2-1/2" square (4)	110	21	17	13	11
	Saltines 2" square (4)	50	10	8	6	5
	Hamburger, with bun (1 burger)	409	78	63	48	41
	meat only (1 patty)	185	36	28	22	19
	Hot dogs (1)	170	33	26	20	17
	Peanuts (1/4 cup) or peanut butter (2 tbsp)	200	38	30	23	20
	Pizza, cheese only (1 5-1/2" sector)	185	36	28	22	19
	sausage and cheese (1 5-1/2" sector)	315	61	48	37	32
	Popcorn plain (2 cups)	80	15	12	9	8
	butter and salt (2 cups)	150	29	23	18	15
	Potato chips (1 cup)	230	44	35	27	23
	Turnover, any fruit flavour (1)	410	79	63	48	41
	Walnuts (1/4 cup)	162	31	25	19	16

Number of minutes of exercise required to expend the caloric energy of the food items shown below

		Food Energy Calories	1) Walking (min)	2) Bicycling (min)	3) Swimming (min)	4) Jogging (min)
Seafood	Cod, fried in butter (4 oz)	162	31	25	19	16
	Haddock, fried, breaded (3 oz)	140	27	22	16	14
	Halibut, grilled with butter (3 oz)	146	28	22	17	15
	Herring (1 herring)	217	42	33	26	22
	Lobster, canned (3 oz)	150	29	23	18	15
	Mackerel, cooked (3 oz)	200	38	31	24	20
	Ocean perch, breaded, fried (3 oz)	195	38	30	23	20
	Salmon, canned (3 oz)	120	23	18	14	12
	fresh, fried (3 oz)	155	30	24	18	16
	Sardines (3 oz)	175	34	27	21	18
	Sole, fillet in butter (3 oz)	172	33	26	20	17
	Tuna (3 oz)	170	33	26	20	17
Vegetables	Asparagus, cooked (1/2 cup)	15	3	2	2	2
	Beans, baked with pork and					
	tomato sauce (1/2 cup)	155	29	24	18	16
	kidney (1/2 cup)	115	22	18	14	12
	snap (yellow or green) (1/2 cup)	15	3	2	2	2
	Beets, cooked (1/2 cup)	28	5	4	3	3
	Broccoli (1/2 cup)	20	4	3	2	2
	Brussels sprouts (1/2 cup)	28	5	4	3	3
	Cabbage, raw (1/2 cup)	10	2	2	1	1
	cooked (1/2 cup)	18	3	3	2	2
	Carrots, raw (1) or cooked (1/2 cup)	20	4	3	2	2
	Cauliflower (3/4 cup)	196	37	30	23	20
	Celery (1 stalk)	5	1	1	1	1
	Coleslaw (1/2 cup)	99	19	15	12	10
	Corn, whole cob (1 ear), kernels,					
	cooked or canned (1/2 cup)	70	13	11	8	7
	Cucumbers (6 slices)	5	1	1	1	1
	Eggplant (1/2 cup)	19	4	3	2	2
	Lettuce, leaves (2 large)	10	2	2	1	1
	Mixed vegetables (1/2 cup)	51	10	8	6	5
	Peas, cooked (1/2 cup)	58	11	9	7	6
	dried, cooked (1/2 cup)	145	28	22	17	14
	Peppers, raw or cooked (1 pod)	15	3	2	2	2
	Potatoes, boiled or baked (1)	80	15	12	9	8
	French fries (10)	155	30	24	18	16
	mashed (1/2 cup)	93	18	14	11	9
	Spinach (1/2 cup)	20	4	3	2	2
	Squash, summer (1/2 cup)	15	3	2	2	2
	winter (1/2 cup)	65	12	10	8	6
	Tomatoes, raw (1 med.), canned or juice (3/4 cup)	35	7	5	4	4
	Turnips (1/2 cup)	35	7	5	4	4
Miscellaneous	Butter (1 pat)	35	7	5	4	4
	Cashew nuts (1/4 cup)	196	37	30	23	20
	Cheeses					
	Cheddar (1" cube - 1 oz)	116	22	18	14	12
	Cottage, creamed - 4% fat (1/2 cup)	120	23	18	14	12
	Cheddar, processed (1 oz)	105	20	16	12	10
	Cottage, not creamed (1/2 cup)	85	16	13	10	8
	Cream (1 oz/2 tbsp)	105	20	16	12	10
	Jams, jellies and preserves (2 tbsp)	110	21	17	13	11
	Soups, cream type made with milk only (3/4 cup)	100	19	16	12	10
	Sugar (1 tbsp)	40	8	6	5	4
	Syrups, table blend or maple (1 tbsp)	60	12	9	7	6
	Yogurt, made from partially skimmed milk (6 oz)	112	22	17	13	11

1 Walking briskly at 3.5 to 4.0 m.p.h. at an average cost of 5.2 cal./minute. The calorie cost will vary according to body weight, type of shoe, type of surface and the terrain.

2 Bicycling at around 6.5 cal./minute (about 7 m.p.h.). The calorie cost will vary depending upon the terrain, type of surface, type of bicycle, speed, efficiency and skill.

3 Swimming at an average of 30 yards/minute, consuming approximately 8.5 cal./minute. A poor swimmer will use more calories.

4 Jogging alternating with walking (5 minutes jogging and 5 minutes walking) will expend around 10 cal./minute.

Dial-a-Power Food Directory

Note: All items in this directory are recommended unless otherwise indicated. Most can be obtained from your local supermarket or general food store. Those only abailable from health food stores or pharmacies are followed by an asterisk*. Those not recommended are followed by (NR).

POWER FOOD

K

L

M

O

P

R

S